# The Ultimate Comfort Food Guide For A Tasty Lunch

Super simple cookbook for everyday comfort food meals

Lawrence Mead

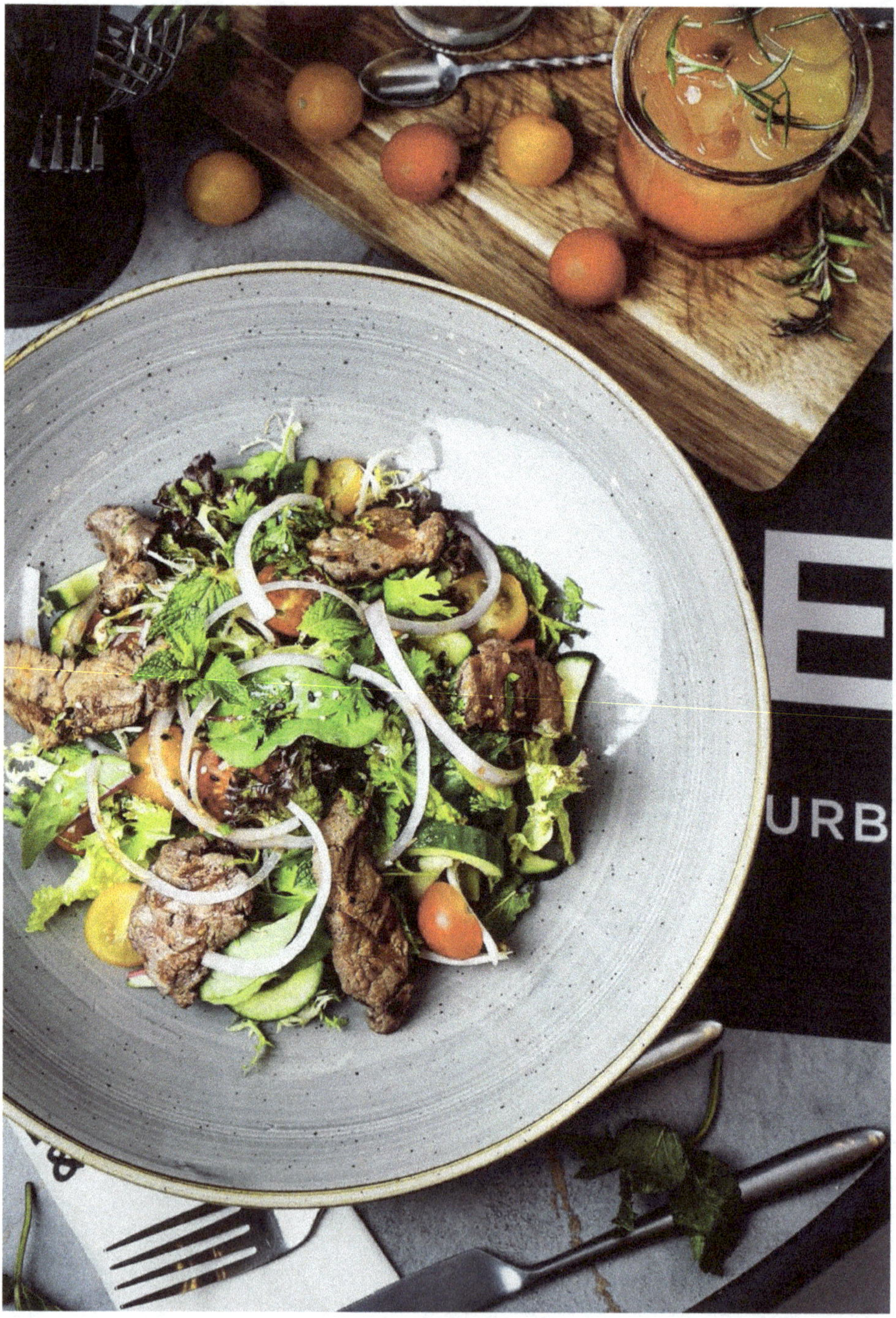
URB

incurred as a result of the use of information contained within this document, including, but not limited to, — errors, omissions, or inaccuracies.

## Table of Contents

# Fennel Chicken

Preparation Time: 10 minutes | Cooking Time: 15 minutes | Servings: 4

**Ingredients:**

1 lb chicken thighs, boneless and cut into three pieces

1 tsp cayenne

1 tsp turmeric

1 tsp garam masala

1 tsp ground fennel seeds

1 tsp paprika

2 tsp garlic, minced

2 tsp ginger, minced

1 tbsp olive oil

1 onion, sliced

Pepper

Salt

**Directions:**

Add chicken and remaining ingredients into the mixing bowl and toss well and place it in the refrigerator overnight.

Spray Pressure Pot multi-level air fryer basket with cooking spray.

Add marinated chicken mixture into the air fryer basket and place basket into the Pressure Pot.

Seal pot with air fryer lid and select air fry mode then set the temperature to 360° F and timer for 15 minutes. Mix halfway through.

Serve and enjoy.

**Nutrition:**

Calories 281, Fat 14.2g, Carbohydrates 0.7g, Sugar 0g, Protein 33g, Cholesterol 116mg.

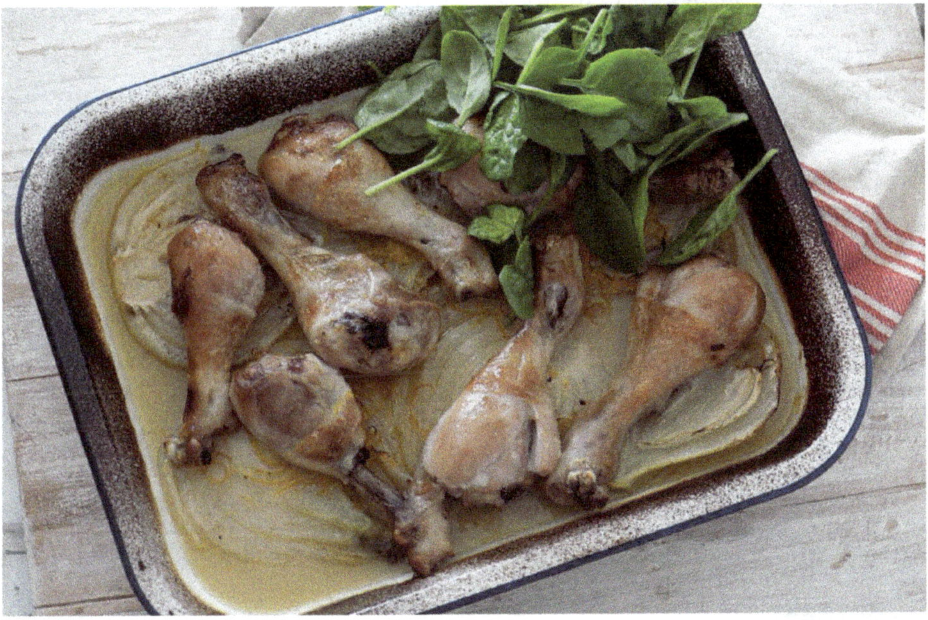

# Beef Pot Roast

Preparation time: 10 minutes | Cooking Time: 1 hour | Servings: 6

**Ingredients:**

3 pounds beef roast

Salt and ground black pepper, to taste

17 ounces beef stock

3 ounces red wine

½ teaspoon chicken salt

½ teaspoon smoked paprika

1 yellow onion, peeled and chopped

4 garlic cloves, peeled and minced

3 carrots, peeled and chopped

5 potatoes, chopped

**Directions:**

In a bowl, mix the salt, pepper, chicken, salt, and paprika and stir.

Rub the beef with this mixture and put it into the Pressure Pot.

Add the onion, garlic, stock, and wine, toss to coat, cover the Pressure Pot and cook on Meat Stew for 50 minutes.

Release the pressure, uncover the Pressure Pot, add the carrots and potatoes, cover again, and cook on the Steam setting for 10 minutes.

Release the pressure again, uncover the Pressure Pot, transfer the roast to a platter, drizzle cooking juices all over, and serve with the vegetables on the side.

**Nutrition:**

Calories 290, Fat 20g, Fiber 0g, Carbs 2g, Protein 25g.

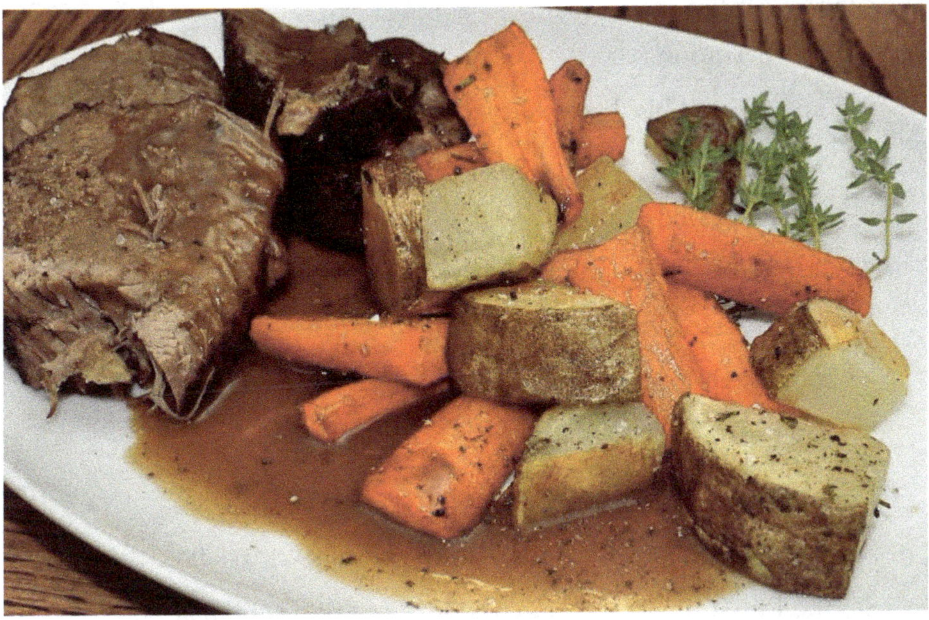

## Beef and Vegetables

Preparation time: 10 minutes | Cooking Time: 30 minutes | Servings: 4

**Ingredients:**

2 tablespoons extra virgin olive oil

1½ pounds, beef chuck roast, cubed

4 tablespoons flour

1 yellow onion, peeled and chopped

2 tablespoons red wine

2 garlic cloves, peeled and minced

2 cups of water

2 cups beef stock

Salt and ground black pepper, to taste

1 bay leaf

½ teaspoon dried thyme

2 celery stalks, chopped

2 carrots, peeled and chopped

4 potatoes, chopped

½ bunch parsley, chopped

**Directions:**

Season the beef with salt and pepper and mix with half of the flour.

Set the Pressure Pot on Sauté mode, add the oil and heat it.

Add the beef, brown for 2 minutes, and transfer to a bowl.

Add the onion to the Pressure Pot, stir, and cook for 3 minutes.

Add the garlic, stir, and cook for 1 minute.

Add the wine, stir well, and cook for 15 seconds. Add the rest of the flour and stir well for 2 minutes.

Return the meat to the Pressure Pot, add the stock, water, bay leaf, and thyme, stir, cover, and cook on the Meat/Stew setting for 12 minutes.

Release the pressure, uncover the Pressure Pot, add the carrots, celery, and potatoes, stir, cover the Pressure Pot, and cook on the Steam setting for 5 minutes.

Release the pressure naturally for 10 minutes, uncover the Pressure Pot, divide among plates, and serve with parsley sprinkled on top.

**Nutrition:**

Calories 221, Fat 5.3g, Fiber 1g, Carbs 20.2g, Protein: 22.7g.

# Trout and Eggplant Mix

Preparation time: 10 minutes | Cooking Time: 15 minutes | Servings: 4

**Ingredients:**

4 trout fillets, boneless

2 scallions, chopped

2 eggplants, cubed

½ cup chicken stock

2 tablespoons parsley, chopped

3 tablespoons olive oil

A pinch of salt and black pepper

2 tablespoons smoked paprika

**Directions:**

Set the Pressure Pot on Sauté mode, add the oil, heat it, add the scallions and the eggplant and cook for 2 minutes,

Add the rest of the ingredients except the parsley, put the lid on, and cook on High for 13 minutes.

Release the pressure naturally for 10 minutes, divide the mix between plates and serve with the parsley sprinkled on top.

**Nutrition:**

Calories 291, fat 16.8g, fiber 4.5g, carbs 6.4g, protein 20g.

# Salmon and Tomato Passata

Preparation time: 10 minutes | Cooking Time: 15 minutes | Servings: 4

**Ingredients:**

1 tablespoon olive oil

4 salmon fillets, boneless, skinless, and cubed

1 tablespoon rosemary, chopped

1 shallot, chopped

1 cup tomato passata

1 teaspoon chili powder

1 tablespoon chives, chopped

A pinch of salt and black pepper

**Directions:**

Set the Pressure Pot on Sauté mode, add the oil, heat it, add the shallot and sauté for 2 minutes.

Add the rest of the ingredients, put the lid on, and cook on High for 12 minutes.

Release the pressure naturally for 10 minutes, divide the mix between plates and serve.

**Nutrition:**

Calories 291, fat 16.8g, fiber 4.5g, carbs 7.4g, protein 20g.

# Salmon and Artichokes

Preparation time: 10 minutes | Cooking Time: 15 minutes | Servings: 4

**Ingredients:**

1 pound salmon, skinless, boneless, and cubed

2 spring onions, chopped

12 ounces canned artichokes, roughly chopped

1 and ½ cups chicken stock

A pinch of salt and black pepper

1 tablespoon cilantro, chopped

**Directions:**

In your Pressure Pot, combine all the ingredients, put the lid on, and cook on High for 15 minutes.

Release the pressure naturally for 10 minutes, divide everything between plates and serve.

**Nutrition:**

Calories 193, fat 7.1g, fiber 4.1g, carbs 6.4g, protein 24.5g.

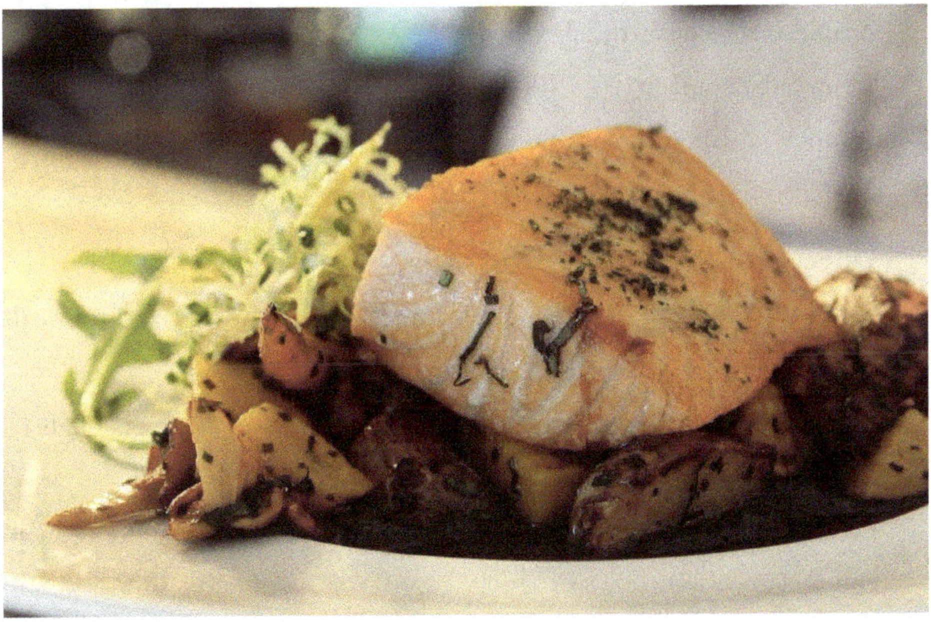

# Trout and Spinach Mix

Preparation time: 5 minutes | Cooking Time: 15 minutes | Servings: 4

**Ingredients:**

6 trout fillets, boneless

2 tablespoons avocado oil

2 scallions, minced

2 garlic cloves, minced

2 tablespoons cilantro, chopped

1 cup baby spinach

A pinch of salt and black pepper

2 tablespoons balsamic vinegar

**Directions:**

Set the Pressure Pot on Sauté mode, add the oil, heat it, add the scallions and the garlic and sauté for 2 minutes.

Add the rest of the ingredients, put the lid on, and cook on High for 12 minutes.

Release the pressure fast for 5 minutes, divide the mix between plates and serve.

**Nutrition:**

Calories 194, fat 8.8g, fiber 0.7g, carbs 1.8g, protein 25.4g.

# Sea Bass and Sauce

Preparation time: 10 minutes | Cooking Time: 15 minutes | Servings: 4

**Ingredients:**

4 sea bass fillets, boneless and skinless

2 tablespoons lime juice

2 garlic cloves, minced

1 shallot, chopped

1 cup chicken stock

1 cup tomato passata

A pinch of salt and black pepper

**Directions:**

In your Pressure Pot, combine the fish with the rest of the ingredients, put the lid on, and cook on High for 15 minutes.

Release the pressure naturally for 10 minutes, divide the mix between plates and serve.

**Nutrition:**

Calories 154, fat 2.9g, fiber 1.3g, carbs 2.5g, protein 25g.

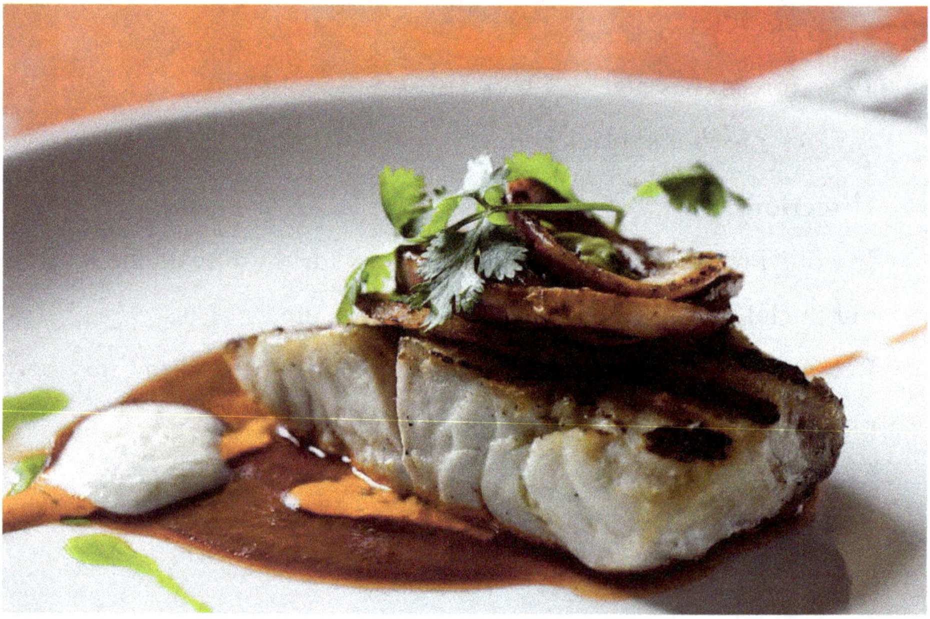

# Sea Bass and Pesto

Preparation time: 5 minutes | Cooking Time: 12 minutes | Servings: 4

**Ingredients:**

4 sea bass fillets, skinless, boneless

2 tablespoons olive oil

2 tablespoons garlic, chopped

1 cup basil, chopped

2 tablespoons pine nuts

A pinch of salt and black pepper

1 cup tomato passata

1 tablespoon parsley, chopped

**Directions:**

In your blender, combine the oil with the garlic, basil, pine nuts, salt, and pepper and pulse well.

In your Pressure Pot, combine the sea bass with the pesto, salt, pepper, tomato passata, and parsley, put the lid on, and cook on High for 12 minutes.

Release the pressure fast for 5 minutes, divide the mix between plates and serve.

**Nutrition:**

Calories 237, fat 12.7g, fiber 1.3g, carbs 5.5g, protein 25.8g.

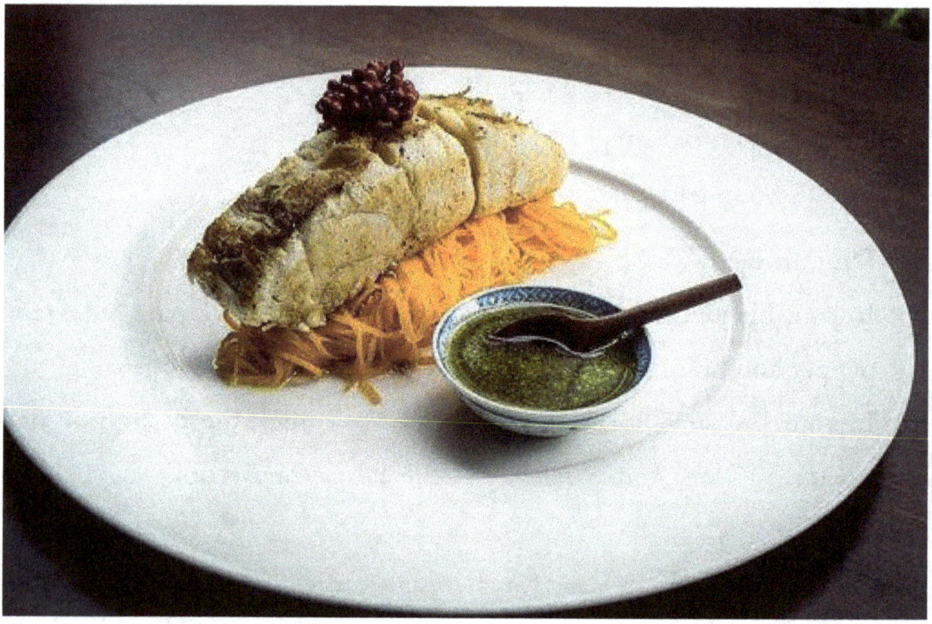

# Tuna and Mustard Greens

Preparation time: 10 minutes | Cooking Time: 10 minutes | Servings: 4

**Ingredients:**

2 cups mustard greens

1 tablespoon olive oil

1 cup tomato passata

1 shallot, chopped

1 tablespoon basil, chopped

A pinch of salt and black pepper

14 ounces tuna fillets, boneless, skinless, and cubed

**Directions:**

Set your Pressure Pot on Sauté mode, add the oil, heat it, add the shallot and sauté for 2 minutes.

Add rest of the ingredients, put the lid on, and cook on High for 8 minutes.

Release the pressure naturally for 10 minutes, divide the mix between plates and serve.

**Nutrition:**

Calories 124, fat 3.7g, fiber 1.9g, carbs 2.6g, protein 1.6g.

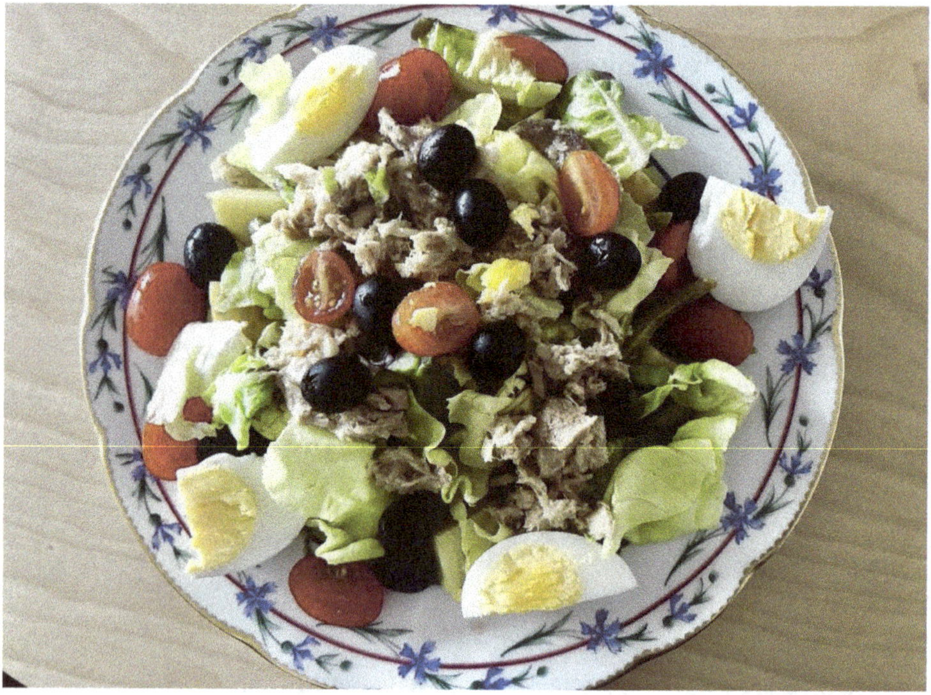

# Salmon and Salsa

Preparation time: 10 minutes | Cooking Time: 8 minutes | Servings: 4

**Ingredients:**

4 salmon fillets, boneless

½ cup veggie stock

1 cup black olives, pitted

1 cup tomatoes, cubed

1 tablespoon basil, chopped

1 tablespoon olive oil

1 tablespoon balsamic vinegar

A pinch of salt and black pepper

1 tablespoon chives, chopped

**Directions:**

In your Pressure Pot, combine the fish with the stock, salt, and pepper put the lid on, and cook on High for 8 minutes.

Release the pressure naturally for 10 minutes and divide the salmon between plates.

In a bowl, mix the olives with the rest of the ingredients, toss, add next to the salmon and serve.

**Nutrition:**

Calories 313, fat 18.2g, fiber 1.7g, carbs 4g, protein 35.4g.

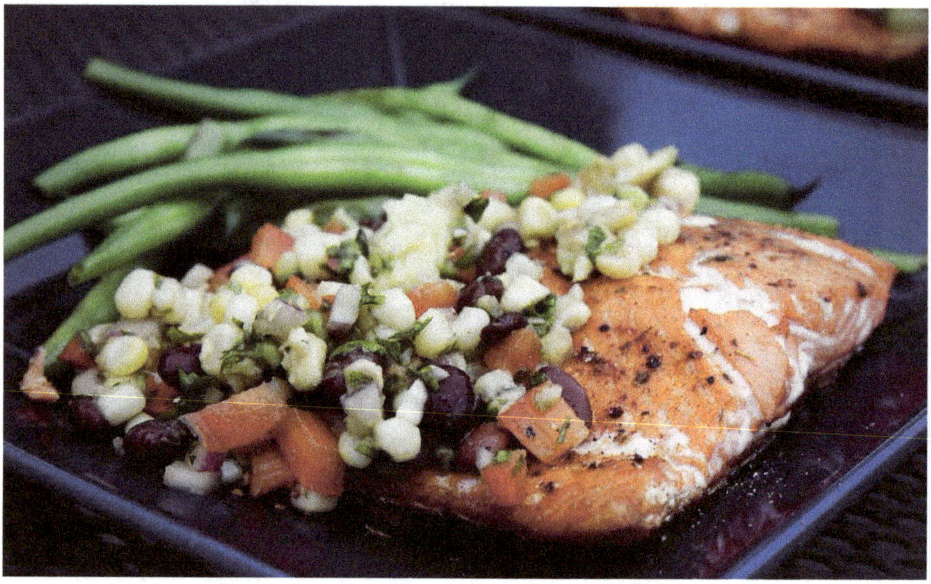

# Moist Cinnamon Muffins

Preparation Time: 10 minutes | Cooking Time: 15 minutes | Servings: 6

**Ingredients:**

1/4 cup pumpkin puree

1/4 cup almond butter

1/4 cup coconut oil

1/2 tbsp cinnamon

1/2 tsp baking powder

1 scoop vanilla protein powder

1/4 cup almond flour

**Directions:**

In a large bowl, mix all dry ingredients.

Add wet ingredients into the dry ingredients and mix until combined.

Pour batter into silicone muffin molds and place into the air fryer basket.

Place basket into the pot.

Seal the pot with an air fryer lid and select bake mode and cook at 350° F for 15 minutes.

Serve and enjoy.

**Nutrition:**

Calories 80, Fat 7.1g, Carbohydrates 1.6g, Sugar 0.4g, Protein 3.5g, Cholesterol 0mg.

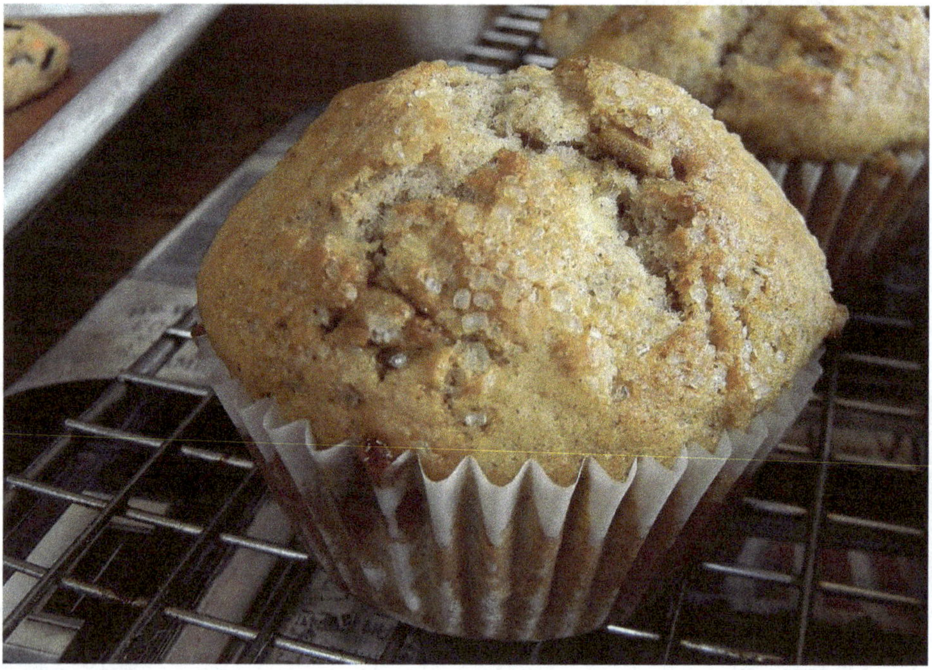

# Meatloaf

Preparation Time: 10 minutes | Cooking Time: 40 minutes | Servings: 8

**Ingredients:**

2 eggs

1/2 cup parmesan cheese, grated

1/2 cup marinara sauce, sugar-free

1 cup cottage cheese

1 lb mozzarella cheese, cut into cubes

2 lbs ground turkey

2 tsp Italian seasoning

1/4 cup basil pesto

1 tsp salt

**Directions:**

Grease Pressure Pot loaf pan with butter and set aside.

Add all ingredients into the mixing bowl and mix until well combined.

Transfer bowl mixture into the prepared loaf pan.

Pour 1/2 cup water into the Pressure Pot and place the steamer rack in the pot.

Place loaf pan on top of the steamer rack.

Seal the pot with an air fryer lid and select bake mode and cook at 400° F for 40 minutes.

Slice and serve.

**Nutrition:**

Calories 350, Fat 18g, Carbohydrates 4.5g, Sugar 1g, Protein 42g, Cholesterol 177mg.

# Bacon Egg Muffins

Preparation Time: 10 minutes | Cooking Time: 25 minutes | Servings: 6

**Ingredients:**

6 eggs

4 bacon slices, cooked and crumbled

1 tbsp fresh parsley, chopped

1/4 tsp mustard powder

1/4 cup heavy cream

2 tbsp green onion, chopped

2 oz cheddar cheese, shredded

Pepper

Salt

**Directions:**

In a bowl, whisk together eggs, mustard powder, heavy cream, pepper, and salt.

Divide cheddar cheese, onions, and bacon into the silicone muffin molds then pour egg mixture into each mold.

Place silicone muffin molds into the Pressure Pot air fryer basket and place the basket in the pot.

Seal the pot with an air fryer lid and select bake mode and cook at 375° F for 25 minutes.

Serve and enjoy.

**Nutrition:**

Calories 116, Fat 8g, Carbohydrates 1g, Sugar 0.5g, Protein 8sg, Cholesterol 178mg.

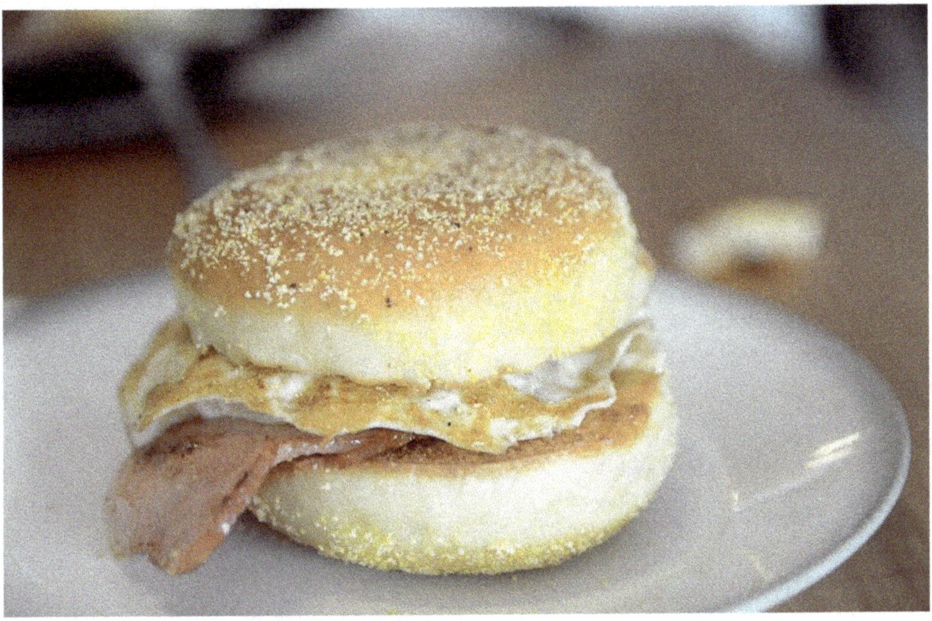

# Zucchini Spinach Muffins

Preparation Time: 10 minutes | Cooking Time: 25 minutes | Servings: 4

**Ingredients:**

2 eggs

1/2 zucchini, grated

1/8 cup parmesan cheese, grated

1/4 cup feta cheese, crumbled

2 tbsp onion spring, chopped

1/4 cup coconut flour

1/8 cup butter, melted

2 tbsp parsley, chopped

1/4 tsp nutmeg

1/8 cup water

1/4 tsp baking powder

1/4 cup spinach, cooked

1/8 tsp black pepper

1/8 tsp salt

**Directions:**

In a bowl, whisk together eggs, water, butter, and salt.

Add baking soda and coconut flour and mix well.

Add onions, nutmeg, parsley, spinach, zucchini, parmesan cheese, feta cheese, pepper, and salt, and stir well.

Pour batter into the silicone muffin molds.

Place silicone muffin molds into the Pressure Pot air fryer basket and place the basket in the pot.

Seal the pot with an air fryer lid and select bake mode and cook at 400° F for 20-25 minutes.

Serve and enjoy.

**Nutrition:**

Calories 236, Fat 18g, Carbohydrates 4g, Sugar 1g, Protein 15g, Cholesterol 135mg.

# Baked Coconut Chicken Wings

Preparation Time: 10 minutes | Cooking Time: 55 minutes | Servings: 4

**Ingredients:**

2 lbs chicken wings

1/8 tsp paprika

2 tsp seasoned salt

1/2 cup coconut flour

1/4 tsp garlic powder

1/2 tsp chili powder

**Directions:**

In a bowl, add all ingredients except chicken wings and mix well.

Add chicken wings to the bowl and toss until well coated.

Line Pressure Pot air fryer basket with parchment paper or foil.

Add chicken wings into the air fryer basket and place the basket in the pot.

Seal the pot with an air fryer lid and select bake mode and cook at 400° F for 55 minutes.

Serve and enjoy.

**Nutrition:**

Calories 440, Fat 17g, Carbohydrates 1g, Sugar 0.2g, Protein 66g, Cholesterol 202mg.

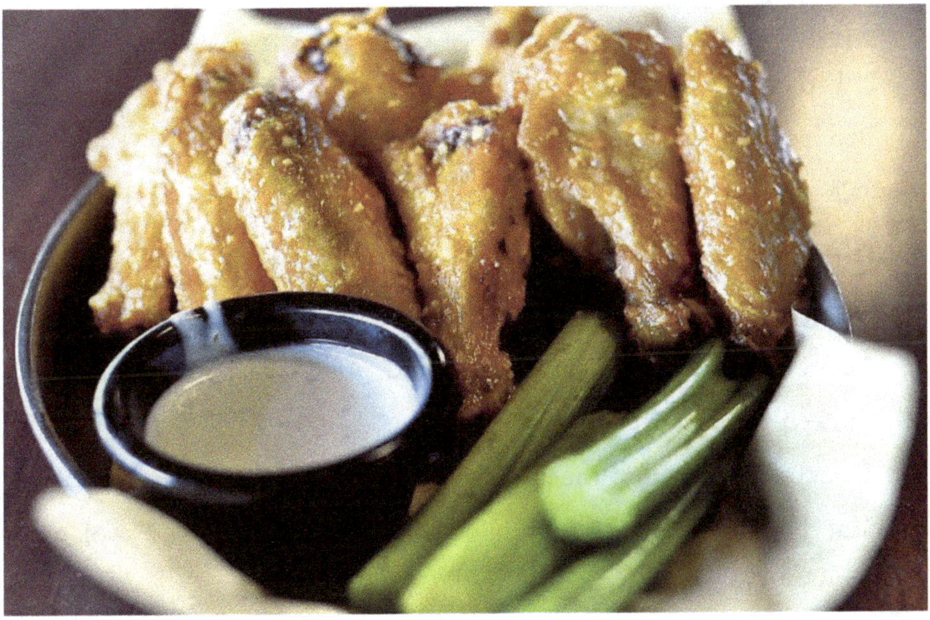

# Butter Garlic Chicken

Preparation Time: 10 minutes | Cooking Time: 40 minutes | Servings: 4

**Ingredients:**

2 lbs chicken drumsticks

1 fresh lemon juice

8 garlic cloves, minced

2 tbsp olive oil

4 tbsp butter, melted

2 tbsp parsley, chopped

Pepper

Salt

**Directions:**

Line Pressure Pot air fryer basket with parchment paper or foil.

Add chicken into the large bowl and pour remaining ingredients over chicken and toss well.

Transfer chicken into the air fryer basket and place basket in the pot.

Seal the pot with an air fryer lid and select bake mode and cook at 400° F for 35-40 minutes.

Serve and enjoy.

**Nutrition:**

Calories 560, Fat 31g, Carbohydrates 3g, Sugar 0.4g, Protein 62g,

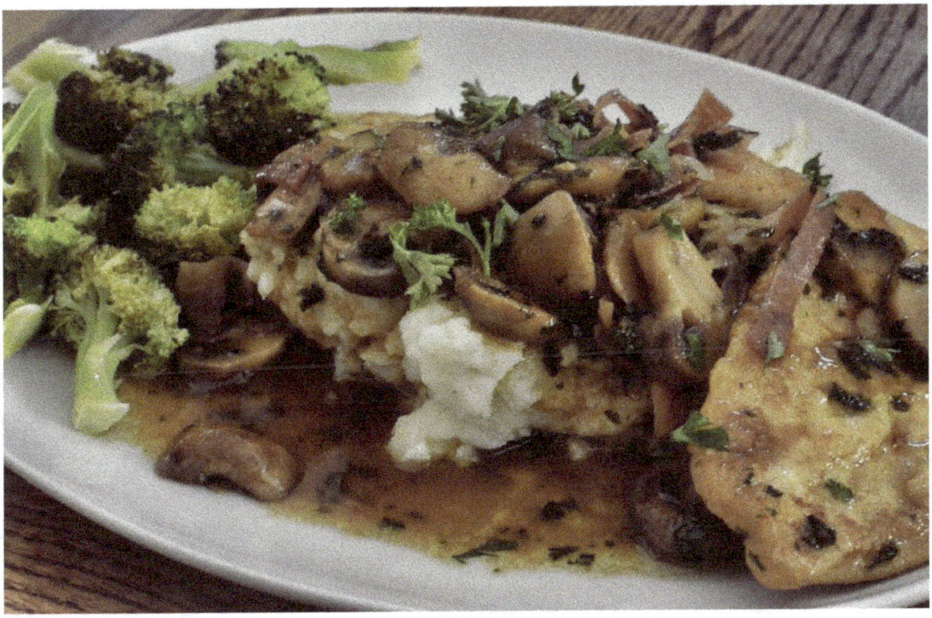

# Crunchy Pecan Crust Chicken

Preparation Time: 10 minutes | Cooking Time: 12 minutes | Servings: 4

**Ingredients:**

1 lb chicken tenders

1 cup pecans, crushed

2 tbsp maple syrup

1/4 cup ground mustard

1/2 tsp paprika

Pepper

Salt

**Directions:**

Season chicken tenders with paprika, pepper, and salt.

Add maple syrup and mustard into the small bowl and mix well.

In a shallow dish, add crushed pecans.

Place the dehydrating tray in a multi-level air fryer basket and place basket in the Pressure Pot.

Brush chicken tenders with maple syrup and coat with crushed pecans and place on dehydrating tray.

Seal pot with air fryer lid and select air fry mode then set the temperature to 350° F and timer for 12 minutes.

Serve and enjoy.

**Nutrition:**

Calories 281, Fat 14.2g, Carbohydrates 0.7g, Sugar 0g, Protein 33g, Cholesterol 116mg.

# Brazilian Chicken Drumsticks

Preparation Time: 10 minutes | Cooking Time: 20 minutes | Servings: 4

**Ingredients:**

1 lb chicken drumsticks

1 tbsp olive oil

1/4 cup lime juice

1/2 tsp cayenne

1/2 tsp coriander seeds, crushed

1/2 tsp black peppercorns, crushed

1 tsp turmeric

1 tsp dried parsley

1 tsp dried oregano

1 tsp cumin seeds

1 tsp salt

**Directions:**

Add chicken drumsticks into the mixing bowl. Add remaining ingredients over chicken and coat well. Place in refrigerator overnight.

Spray Pressure Pot multi-level air fryer basket with cooking spray.

Add marinated chicken drumsticks into the air fryer basket and place the basket into the Pressure Pot.

Seal pot with air fryer lid and select air fry mode then set the temperature to 390° F and timer for 20 minutes. Turn chicken halfway through.

Serve and enjoy.

**Nutrition:**

Calories 281, Fat 14.2g, Carbohydrates 0.7g, Sugar 0g, Protein 33g, Cholesterol 116mg.

# Delicious Chicken Jalfrezi

Preparation Time: 10 minutes | Cooking Time: 15 minutes | Servings: 4

**Ingredients:**

1 lb chicken breasts, boneless and cut into 2-inch pieces

1 tsp cayenne

1 tsp garam masala

1 tsp turmeric

2 tbsp olive oil

2 cups bell pepper, chopped

1 cup onion, chopped

Pepper

Salt

**Directions:**

Add chicken into the large bowl. Add remaining ingredients and toss well.

Spray Pressure Pot multi-level air fryer basket with cooking spray.

Add marinated chicken mixture into the air fryer basket and place basket into the Pressure Pot.

Seal pot with air fryer lid and select air fry mode then set the temperature to 360° F and timer for 15 minutes. Stir halfway through.

Serve and enjoy.

**Nutrition:**

Calories 281, Fat 14.2 g, Carbohydrates 0.7g, Sugar 0g, Protein 33g, Cholesterol 116mg.

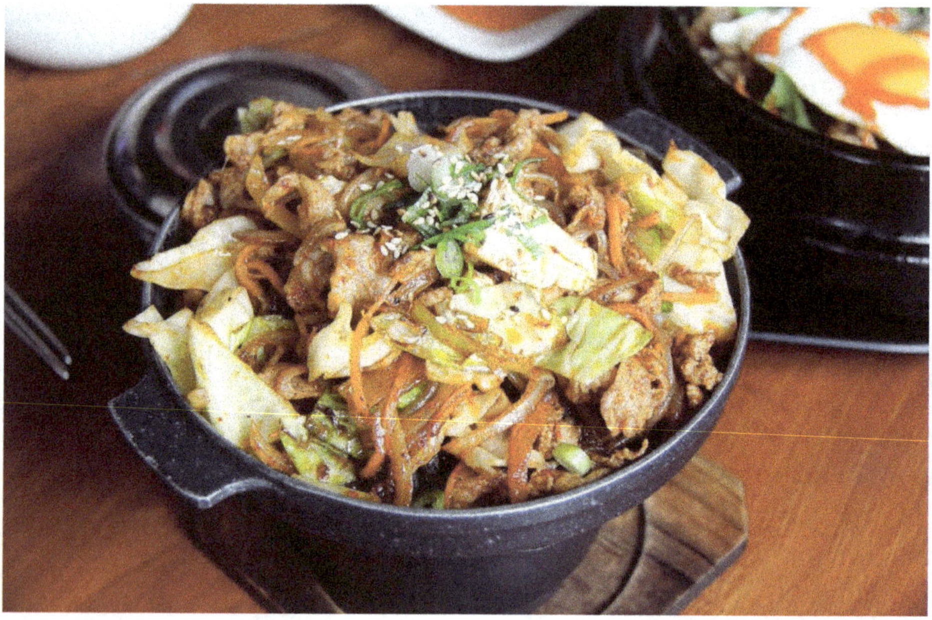

# Roasted Squash

Preparation Time: 10 minutes | Cooking Time: 12 minutes | Servings: 4

**Ingredients:**

1 lb butternut squash, peeled and cut into chunks

1 tsp thyme

1 tbsp sage

1 tbsp olive oil

Pepper

Salt

**Directions:**

Add squash and remaining ingredients into the large bowl and toss well.

Line Pressure Pot multi-level air fryer basket with foil.

Add squash mixture into the air fryer basket and place basket into the Pressure Pot.

Seal pot with air fryer lid and select air fry mode then set the temperature to 390° F and timer for 12 minutes. Stir after 10 minutes.

Serve and enjoy.

**Nutrition:**

Calories 83, Fat 3.7g, Carbohydrates 13.7g, Sugar 2.5g, Protein 1.2g, Cholesterol 0mg.

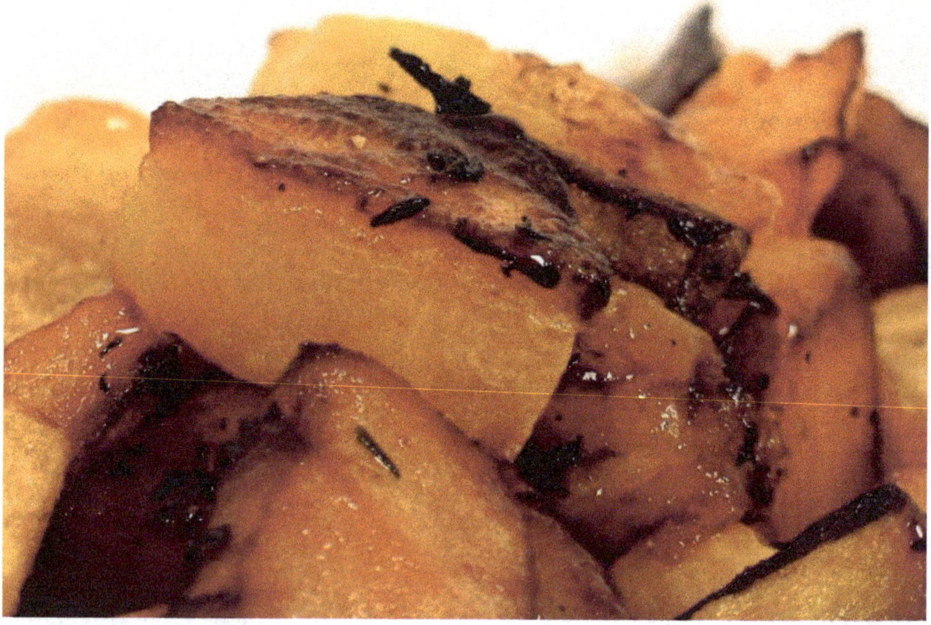

# Balsamic Asparagus

Preparation time: 25 minutes | Cooking Time: 20 minutes | Servings: 4

**Ingredients:**

1 lb. Asparagus stalks

¼ cup olive oil+ 1 tsp.

2 tbsp. Balsamic vinegar

1 tbsp. Lime juice

1 tbsp. Smoked paprika

Salt and black pepper to taste.

**Directions:**

Take a bowl and mix the asparagus with salt, pepper, and 1 tsp. Oil, toss, transfer to your air fryer's basket, and cook at 370°F for 20 minutes.

Meanwhile, in a bowl, mix all the other ingredients and whisk them well

Divide the asparagus between plates, drizzle the balsamic vinaigrette all over and serve as a side dish.

**Nutrition:**

Calories 187, Fat 6g, Fiber 2g, Carbs 4g, Protein 9g.

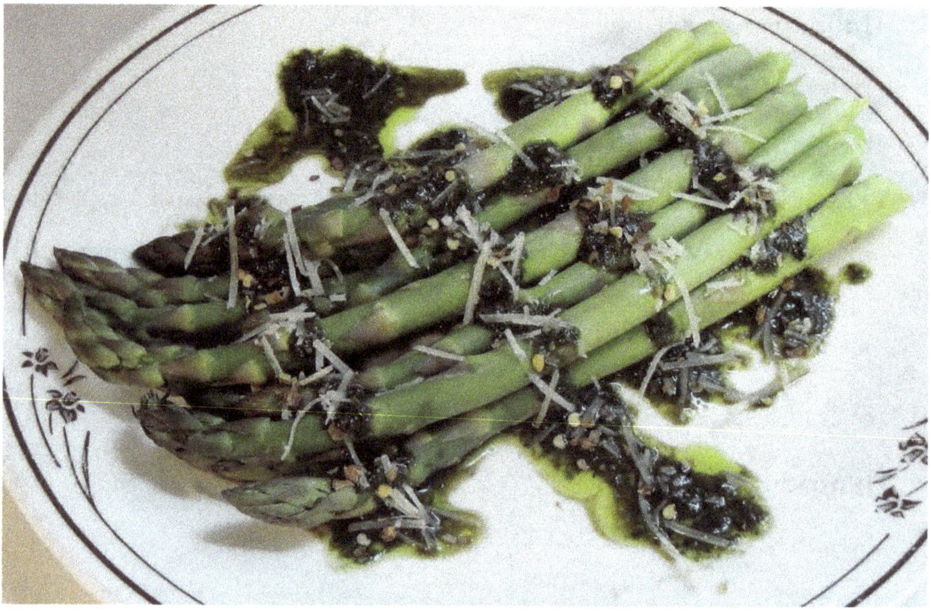

## Zucchini Spaghetti

Preparation time: 20 minutes | Cooking Time: 20 minutes | Servings: 4

**Ingredients:**

1 lb. Zucchinis, cut with a spiralizer

1 cup parmesan; grated

¼ cup parsley; chopped.

¼ cup olive oil

6 garlic cloves; minced

½ tsp. Red pepper flakes

Salt and black pepper to taste.

**Directions:**

In a pan that fits your air fryer, mix all the ingredients , toss, introduce in the fryer and cook at 370°f for 15 minutes

Divide between plates and serve as a side dish.

**Nutrition:**

Calories 200, Fat 6g, Fiber 3g, Carbs 4g, Protein 5g.

# Zucchinis and Walnuts

Preparation time: 25 minutes | Cooking Time: 20 minutes | Servings: 4

**Ingredients:**

1 lb. Zucchinis; sliced

¼ cup chives; chopped.

1 cup walnuts; chopped.

4 oz. Arugula leaves

1 tbsp. Olive oil

Salt and white pepper to the taste

**Directions:**

In a pan that fits the air fryer, combine all the ingredients except the arugula and walnuts, toss, put the pan in the machine, and cook at 360°F for 20 minutes

Transfer this to a salad bowl, add the arugula and the walnuts, toss and serve as a side salad.

**Nutrition:**

Calories 170, Fat 4g, Fiber 1g; Carbs 4g, Protein 5g.

# Tuna Steaks

Preparation Time: 14 minutes | Cooking Time: 5 minutes | Servings: 4

**Ingredients:**

4 medium tuna steaks

1 bunch oregano, fresh

3 tablespoons lemon juice

2 tablespoons soy sauce

1/3 cup white wine

Sea salt and black pepper to taste

Some lettuce and tomatoes for serving

**Directions:**

Place your tuna steaks into your Pressure Pot, add the soy sauce, wine, lemon juice, salt, pepper, and add the steamer basket as well, place the fresh oregano in the steamer basket.

Cook on high for 5minutes.

Release the pressure using the quick-release. Divide the tuna steaks among the serving plates, serve with lettuce and tomatoes on the side.

Serve warm!

**Nutrition:**

Calories 298, Fat 12g, Fiber 2g, Carbs 10g, Protein 26g.

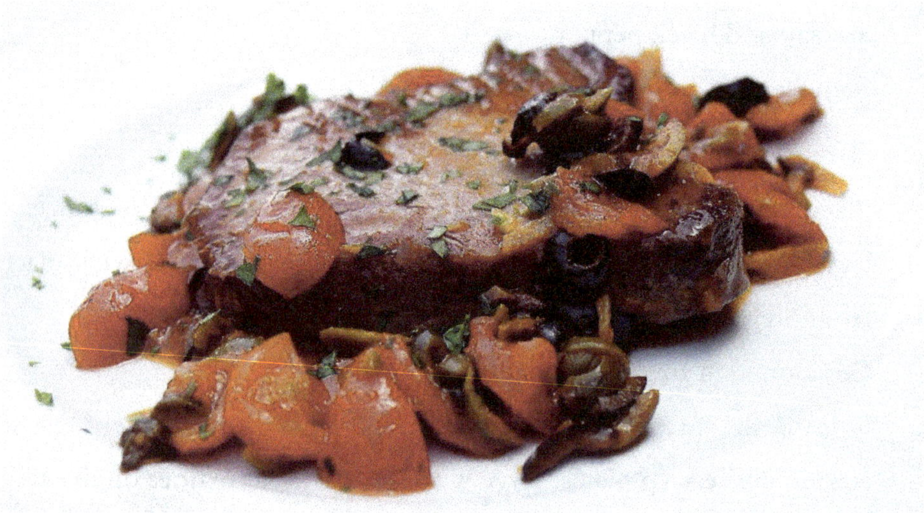

# Chicken Cordon Bleu

Preparation Time: 15 minutes | Cooking Time: 5 minutes | Servings: 2

**Ingredients:**

6 oz chicken fillet

2 ham slices

2 Swiss cheese slices

¼ teaspoon salt

¼ teaspoon white pepper

1 teaspoon butter, melted

½ cup chicken broth

**Directions:**

Beat the chicken fillets with the help of the kitchen hammer to make 2 chicken pieces in the shape of the pancake.

Then brush every chicken piece with melted butter and top with ham and Swiss cheese.

Then sprinkle them with white pepper and salt.

Roll the chicken.

Pour chicken broth into the Pressure Pot.

Place the rolled chicken in the chicken broth and close the lid.

Cook the meal on manual mode (high pressure for 5 minutes.

When the time is over, make a quick pressure release and remove the meal from the Pressure Pot.

**Nutrition:**

Calories 341, fat 18.8g, fiber 0.4g, carbs 3g, protein 38.1g.

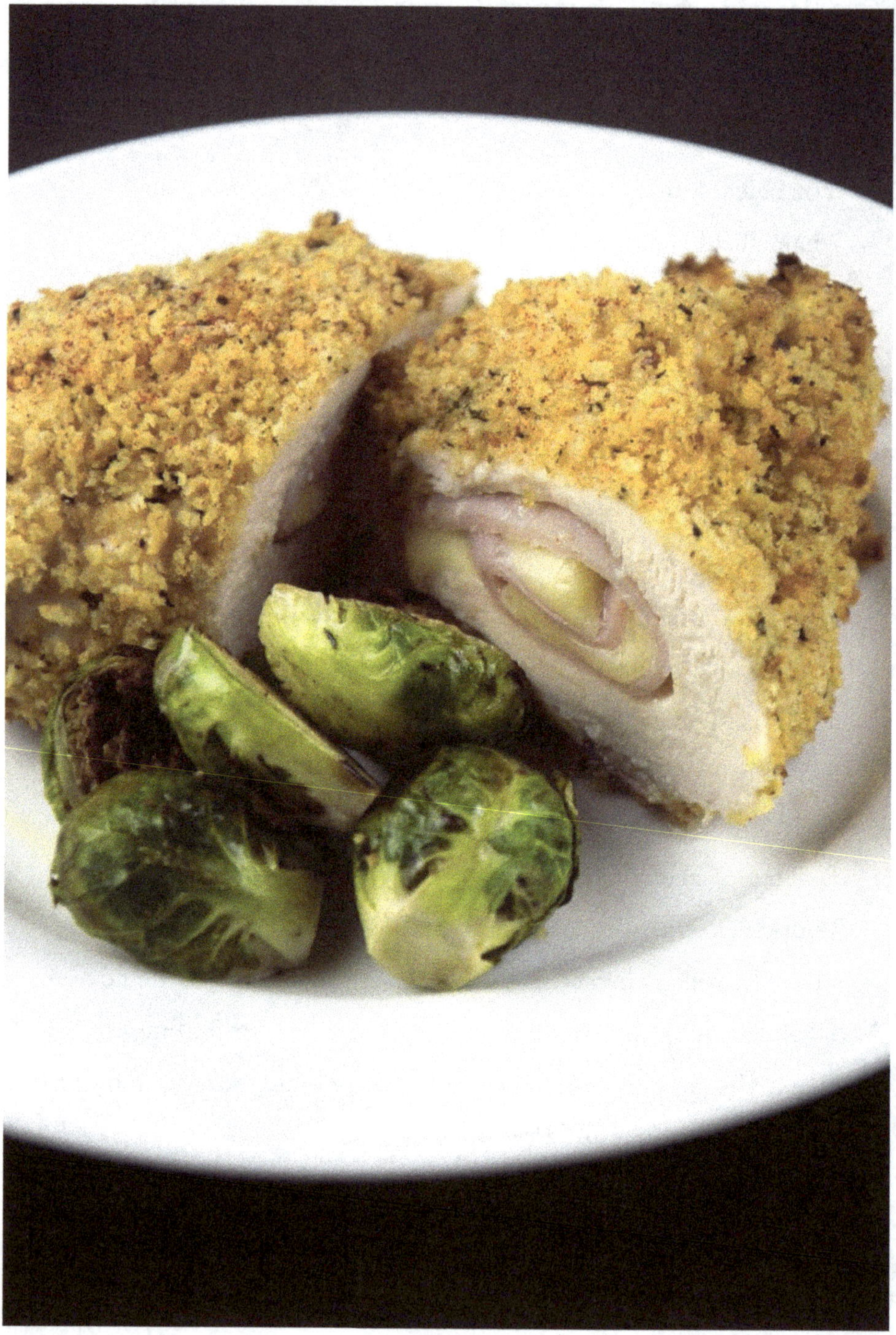

# Herbed Whole Chicken

Preparation Time: 15 minutes | Cooking Time: 50 minutes | Servings: 8

**Ingredients:**

3-pound whole chicken

1 teaspoon ground cumin

½ teaspoon ground nutmeg

1 teaspoon fresh thyme

1 teaspoon fresh rosemary

1 teaspoon smoked paprika

1 teaspoon sage

1 tablespoon fresh basil, chopped

½ teaspoon cayenne pepper

1 teaspoon ground turmeric

1 teaspoon onion powder

¼ cup sesame oil

1 teaspoon dried oregano

1 teaspoon salt

3 garlic cloves, peeled

1 ½ cup water, for cooking

**Directions:**

Pour water into the Pressure Pot and add garlic cloves.

Then insert the trivet.

In the mixing bowl combine sesame oil with all spices and herbs from the list above.

Rub the chicken with oil mixture well and place it in the Pressure Pot (on the trivet).

Close the lid and set manual mode (high pressure).

Cook the chicken for 50 minutes.

When the time is over, allow the natural pressure release for 10 minutes.

**Nutrition:**

Calories 472, fat 35.5g, fiber 0.5g, carbs 1.5g, protein 35.5g.

# Ground Chicken Mix

Preparation Time: 10 minutes | Cooking Time: 14 minutes | Servings: 3

**Ingredients:**

8 oz ground chicken

2 medium celery stalks, chopped

2 oz fennel, chopped

½ teaspoon ground black pepper

1 teaspoon smoked paprika

1 tablespoon cream cheese

1 teaspoon coconut oil

1/3 teaspoon salt

**Directions:**

Place the coconut oil in the Pressure Pot and melt it.

Add celery stalk and fennel. Cook the vegetables for 4 minutes on sauté mode. Stir them after 2 minutes of cooking.

Meanwhile, in the mixing bowl combine ground chicken, ground black pepper, smoked paprika, and salt.

Add the ground chicken mixture in the Pressure Pot and cook on sauté mode for 3 minutes.

After this, add cream cheese, stir well and close the lid.

Cook the ground chicken mix for 7 minutes more.

**Nutrition:**

Calories 181, fat 8.5g, fiber 1.4g, carbs 2.9g, protein 22.7g.

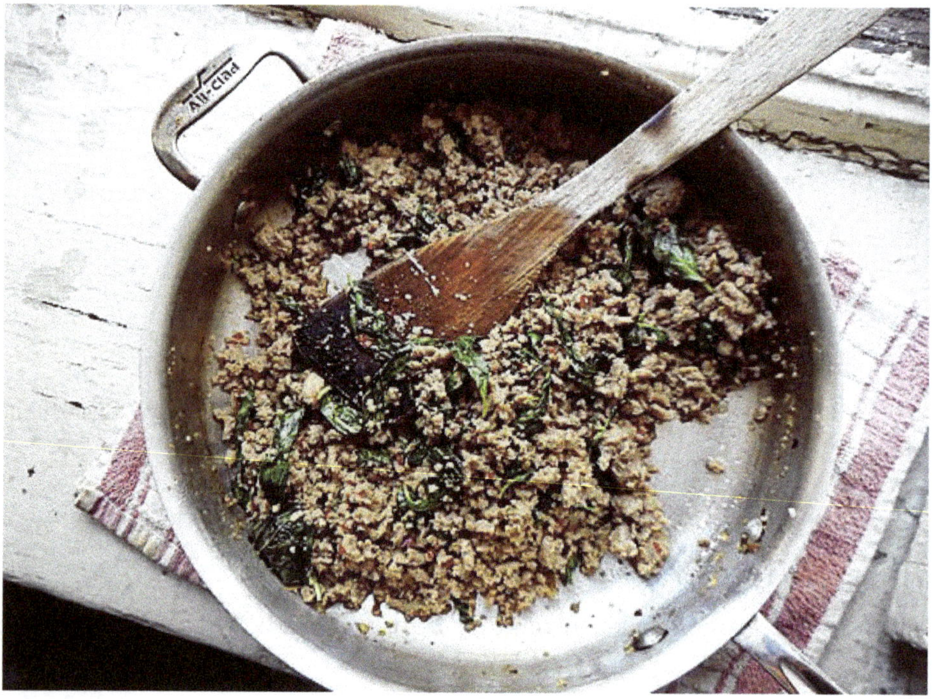
All-Clad

# Bacon-Wrapped Chicken Tenders

Preparation Time: 15 minutes | Cooking Time: 14 minutes | Servings: 6

**Ingredients:**

10 oz chicken breast, skinless, boneless

3 bacon slices

¼ teaspoon salt

¼ teaspoon ground black pepper

¼ teaspoon ground turmeric

1 cup water, for cooking

**Directions:**

Rub the chicken breast with ground black pepper, ground turmeric, and salt.

Pour water and insert trivet in the Pressure Pot.

Arrange the chicken breast on the trivet and close the lid.

Cook it on manual mode (high pressure for 10 minutes.

When the time is over, make a quick pressure release and remove the chicken from the Pressure Pot.

Shred-it with the help of the fork and knife.

After this, clean the Pressure Pot and remove the trivet.

Cut every bacon slice into halves.

Place the bacon halves in the Pressure Pot and cook on sauté mode for 2 minutes from each side.

After this, make the small tenders from the shredded chicken mixture with the help of the fingertips.

Then wrap every tender in the cooked bacon and secure with the toothpick.

**Nutrition:**

Calories 106, fat 5.2g, fiber 0g, carbs 0.3g, protein 13.6g.

## Chicken and Spinach Bowl

Preparation Time: 10 minutes | Cooking Time: 15 minutes | Servings: 4

**Ingredients:**

10 oz chicken fillet, chopped

½ teaspoon paprika

¼ teaspoon salt

¼ teaspoon ground black pepper

½ teaspoon cayenne pepper

1 tablespoon sesame oil

1 red onion, sliced

1 cup fresh spinach, chopped

¼ cup of water

**Directions:**

Heat Pressure Pot on sauté mode for 3 minutes.

In the mixing bowl combine paprika, salt, chicken fillet, ground black pepper, ½ tablespoon of sesame oil, and cayenne pepper.

Shake the ingredients gently and place them in the Pressure Pot.

Close the lid and sauté them for 5 minutes.

Then stir the chicken well and add water.

Close the lid and sauté it for 10 minutes more.

Meanwhile, mix up together spinach and red onion. Add remaining sesame oil.

Place the spinach mixture in the serving bowls and top them with cooked chicken.

**Nutrition:**

Calories 179, fat 8.8g, fiber 1g, carbs 3.2g, protein 21.1g.

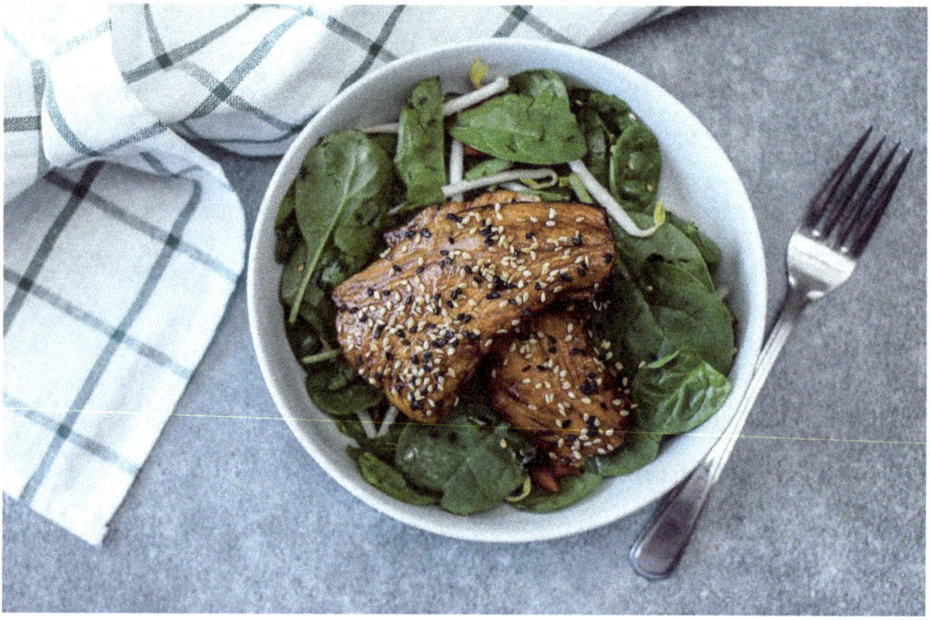

# Keto Chicken Burger

Preparation Time: 10 minutes | Cooking Time: 10 minutes | Servings: 2

**Ingredients:**

½ cup ground chicken

1 tomato, sliced

4 lettuce leaves

¼ teaspoon cayenne pepper

1 teaspoon dried dill

½ teaspoon onion powder

¼ teaspoon garlic powder

1 tablespoon almond meal

¼ teaspoon salt

1 cup water, for cooking

**Directions:**

Pour water and insert the trivet in the Pressure Pot.

In the mixing bowl combine ground chicken with cayenne pepper, dried dill, onion powder, garlic powder, salt, and almond meal.

Stir the ground mixture until smooth.

Then make 2 balls from the ground chicken mixture, press them gently in the shape of a burger and place them in the trivet.

Close the lid and cook the chicken balls for 10 minutes on manual mode (high pressure).

When the time is over, make a quick pressure release.

Place the chicken balls on 2 lettuce leaves.

Top them with sliced tomato and remaining lettuce leaves.

**Nutrition:**

Calories 96, fat 4.2g, fiber 1g, carbs 3.3g, protein 11.3g.

# Chicken Liver Pate

Preparation Time: 15 minutes | Cooking Time: 8 minutes | Servings: 8

**Ingredients:**

2-pound chicken liver

1/3 cup butter, softened

½ white onion, diced

½ teaspoon salt

½ teaspoon ground black pepper

½ teaspoon dried oregano

1 cup water, for cooking

**Directions:**

Put 1 tablespoon of butter in the Pressure Pot and melt it on sauté mode for 3 minutes.

After this, add diced onion and cook it for 5 minutes or until it is golden brown.

Then transfer the onion to the big bowl and clean the Pressure Pot.

Pour water and insert the trivet in the Pressure Pot.

Mix up together chicken liver with salt and ground black pepper.

Place the liver on the trivet (you can line the trivet with baking paper) and close the lid.

Cook the chicken liver on steam mode for 8 minutes.

When the time is over, allow the natural pressure release for 10 minutes and open the lid.

Transfer the chicken liver to the food processor and blend it until smooth.

Then add smooth liver in the onion; add butter and dried oregano.

Stir the paste until homogenous.

Store it in the fridge for up to 7 days.

**Nutrition:**

Calories 261, fat 15.1g, fiber 0.2g, carbs 1.8g, protein 27.9g.

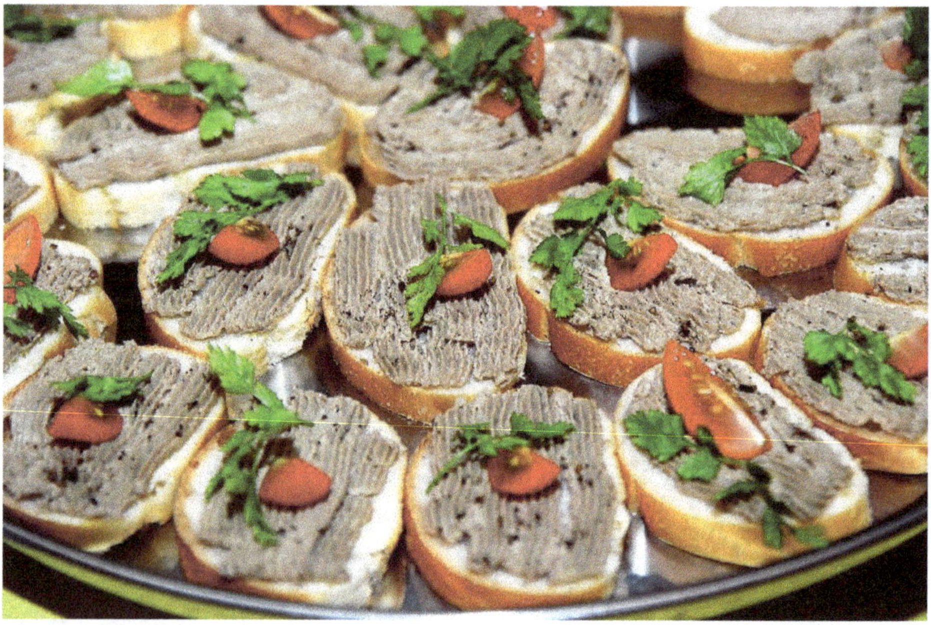

# Coconut Chicken Cubes

Preparation Time: 10 minutes | Cooking Time: 12 minutes | Servings: 3

**Ingredients:**

10 oz chicken fillet

3 tablespoons coconut flakes

2 tablespoons coconut flour

4 tablespoons butter

½ teaspoon salt

½ teaspoon turmeric

½ teaspoon chili powder

2 tablespoons cream cheese

**Directions:**

Chop the chicken fillet into medium cubes.

Then sprinkle them with salt, turmeric, and chili powder.

After this, dip every chicken cube in cream cheese.

In the bowl mix up together coconut flakes and coconut flour.

Coat every chicken cube in the coconut mixture.

Melt butter in the Pressure Pot on sauté mode (appx. 3-4 minutes).

Then arrange the chicken cubes in the hot butter in one layer.

Cook the coconut chicken cubes for 4 minutes and then flip them on another side.

Cook the meal for 4 minutes more.

**Nutrition:**

Calories 379, fat 27g, fiber 2.7g, carbs 4.8g, protein 28.9g.

# Chicken Lettuce Rolls

Preparation Time: 10 minutes | Cooking Time: 11 minutes | Servings: 4

**Ingredients:**

4 lettuce leaves

8 oz chicken, grinded

1 garlic clove, diced

1 teaspoon dried parsley

¼ teaspoon chili flakes

¼ carrot, grated

1 teaspoon coconut oil

1 teaspoon ricotta cheese

1 tablespoon heavy cream

1 teaspoon apple cider vinegar

**Directions:**

In the bowl mix up ground chicken, garlic, parsley, chili flakes, and carrot.

Put the coconut oil in the Pressure Pot.

Set sauté mode and heat it for 1 minute.

Then add chicken mixture.

Cook it on sauté mode for 5 minutes. Stir it from time to time with the help of a spatula.

After this, add heavy cream and ricotta cheese. Stir well.

Add apple cider vinegar. Stir the chicken one more time and cook it for 5 minutes more.

Then fill the lettuce leaves with chicken mixture and roll them in the shape of pockets.

**Nutrition:**

Calories 114, fat 4.4g, fiber 0.2g, carbs 1g, protein 16.8g.

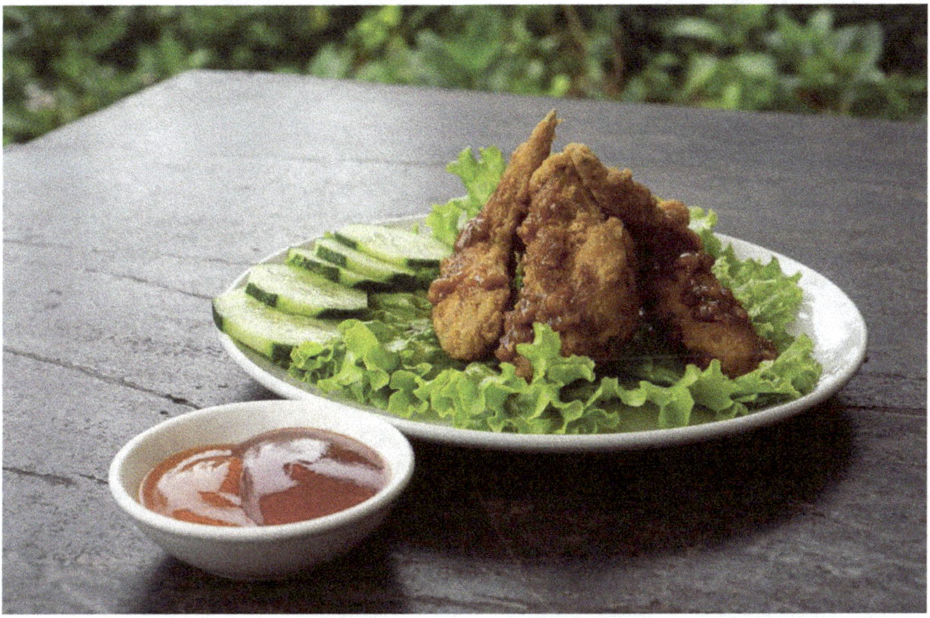

# Turkey Bolognese Sauce

Preparation Time: 10 minutes | Cooking Time: 17 minutes | Servings: 4

**Ingredients:**

¼ cup carrot, grated

½ white onion, minced

1 garlic clove, diced

¼ teaspoon salt

10 oz ground turkey

1/3 teaspoon chili flakes

½ teaspoon dried thyme

1 teaspoon tomato paste

1 oz Swiss cheese, grated

½ scoop stevia powder

1 tablespoon coconut oil

1/3 cup water

**Directions:**

Toss coconut oil in the Pressure Pot and melt it on sauté mode.

Then add carrot, garlic, and onion. Cook the ingredients for 5 minutes. Stir them with the help of the spatula after 3 minutes of cooking.

Then add salt and ground turkey,

Sprinkle the ingredients with chili flakes, dried thyme, and stevia powder. Mix up well and sauté for 3 minutes.

After this, mix up water with tomato paste.

Pour the liquid over the ground turkey. Stir the sauce well and close the lid.

Cook it on manual mode (high pressure for 4 minutes).

When the time is over, make a quick pressure release and open the lid.

Top the sauce with Swiss cheese and mix up until the cheese is melted. The sauce is cooked.

**Nutrition:**

Calories 205, fat 13.2g, fiber 0.6g, carbs 2.9g, protein 21.6g.

# Tuna Casserole

Preparation Time: 14 minutes | Cooking Time: 4 minutes | Servings: 4

**Ingredients:**

2 ½ cups macaroni pasta

10-ounces cream of mushroom soup

14-ounces of canned tuna, drained

1 cup cheddar cheese, shredded

1 cup peas

3 cups of water

Salt and black pepper to taste

**Directions:**

In your Pressure Pot mix the water, mushroom soup, tuna, macaroni, peas, salt, pepper, and stir. Cover and cook on high for 4-minutes.

Release the pressure using the quick-release.

Add the shredded cheese then cover your pot and allow it to sit for 5minutes. Divide among serving bowls.

Serve warm or cold!

**Nutrition:**

Calories 287, Fat 12g, Fiber 2g, Carbs 17g, Protein 28g.

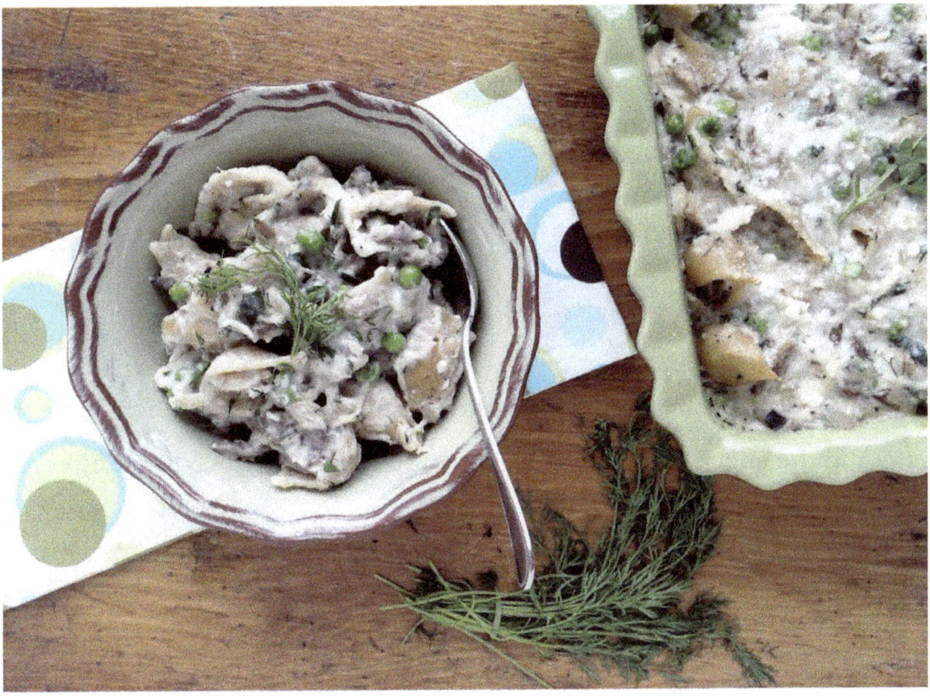

# Zucchini Pasta with Capers

Preparation Time: 14 minutes | Cooking Time: 8 minutes | Servings: 4

**Ingredients:**

2 tablespoons capers

Water

16-ounces of zucchini pasta

11-ounces of canned tuna in oil

3 anchovies

1 tablespoon olive oil

1 garlic clove, minced

2 cups tomato puree

Sea salt to taste

**Directions:**

Set your Pressure Pot to the sauté mode, add the oil and heat it.

Add the anchovies and garlic, stir and sauté them for 2-minutes.

Add tomato puree, tuna, salt, and stir.

Add the water cover and cook for 3-minutes on low.

Release the pressure on quick-release. Divide then place the tuna mix on top of a bed of zucchini pasta and top with capers.

Serve warm!

**Nutrition:**

Calories 267, Fat 7g, Fiber 1g, Carbs 14g, Protein 23g.

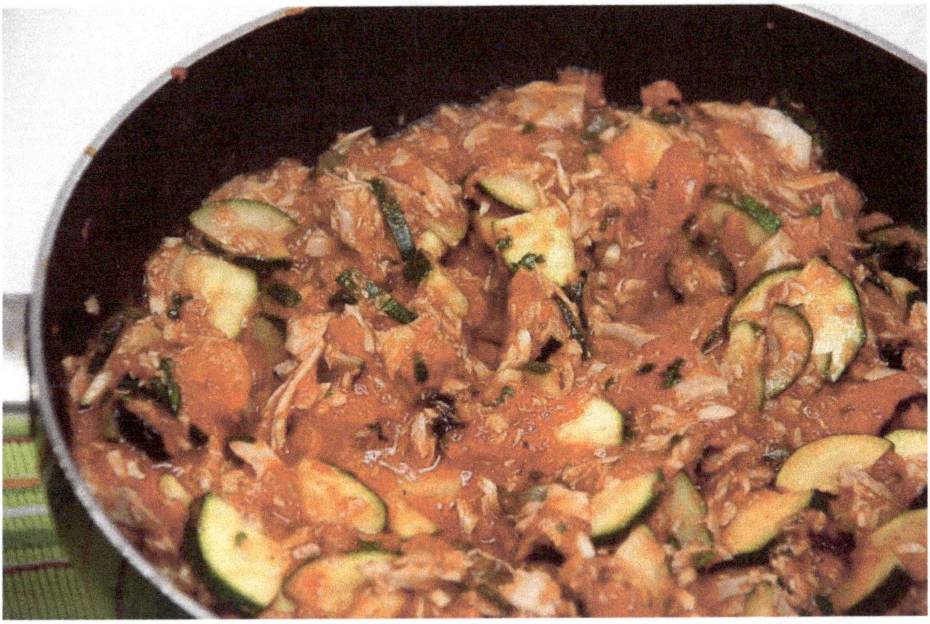

# Beans & Clams

Preparation Time: 14 minutes | Cooking Time: 10 minutes | Servings: 6

**Ingredients:**

10-ounces canned white beans, drained

1 bay leaf

2 garlic cloves, minced

1 tablespoon olive oil

4-ounces white wine

14-ounces clams

A dash of salt

**Directions:**

Place the beans in your Pressure Pot, add water to cover, a pinch of salt, and bay leaf, stir.

Cover and cook on high for 10-minutes.

Release the pressure using quick-release. Drain the beans and clean your pot.

Add the oil and set to sauté mode, and heat the oil.

Add the garlic, stir and cook for 2-minutes.

Add wine, beans, clams, cover, and cook on high for 6-minutes.

Release the pressure again using quick-release.

Divide the clams and beans into serving bowls.

Serve warm!

**Nutrition:**

Calories 254, Fat 6g, Fiber 2g, Carbs 8g, Protein 21g.

# Pressure Pot Squid

Preparation Time: 14 minutes | Cooking Time: 25 minutes | Servings: 4

**Ingredients:**

1 small ginger piece, grated

2 yellow onions, chopped

1 lb. squid, cut into medium pieces

10-garlic cloves, minced

2 green chilies, chopped

3 tablespoons olive oil

¾ cup of water

1 teaspoon mustard seeds

1 teaspoon garam masala

Black pepper to taste

A pinch of sea salt

Pinch of turmeric powder

¾ tablespoon chili powder

½ tablespoon lemon juice

¼ cup coconut, shredded

1 tablespoon coriander, ground

**Directions:**

Place your Pressure Pot on the sauté mode, add the oil and heat it.

Add the mustard seeds, stir and toast them for 1-minute.

Add the coconut, stir, toast for 2-minutes more.

Add the ginger, chilies, onions, garlic, and stir and cook for 1-minute.

Add the curry leaf, pepper, salt, lemon juice, coriander, chili powder, turmeric, garam masala, water, squid, and stir.

Cover and cook on low for 25-minutes.

Release the pressure naturally for 10-minutes.

Divide into serving bowls.

Serve warm!

**Nutrition:**

Calories 241, Fat 12g, Fiber 1g, Carbs 11g, Protein 30g.

# Italian Braised Squid

Preparation Time: 14 minutes | Cooking Time: 20 minutes | Servings: 4

**Ingredients:**

1 lb. peas

1 lb. squid, cut into medium pieces

1 tablespoon olive oil

1 tablespoon white wine

½ lb. tomatoes, crushed

Sea salt and pepper to taste

1 yellow onion, chopped

**Directions:**

Add the oil to your Pressure Pot, set it on sauté mode, and heat the oil.

Add the onion, stir and cook for 3-minutes.

Add the squid and cook for an additional 3-minutes.

Add the wine, tomatoes, peas, pepper, and salt, stir, cover, and cook on high for 15-minutes. Release the pressure naturally for 15-minutes.

Divide among serving plates.

Serve warm!

**Nutrition:**

Calories 212, Fat 16g, Fiber 1g, Carbs 13g, Protein 34g.

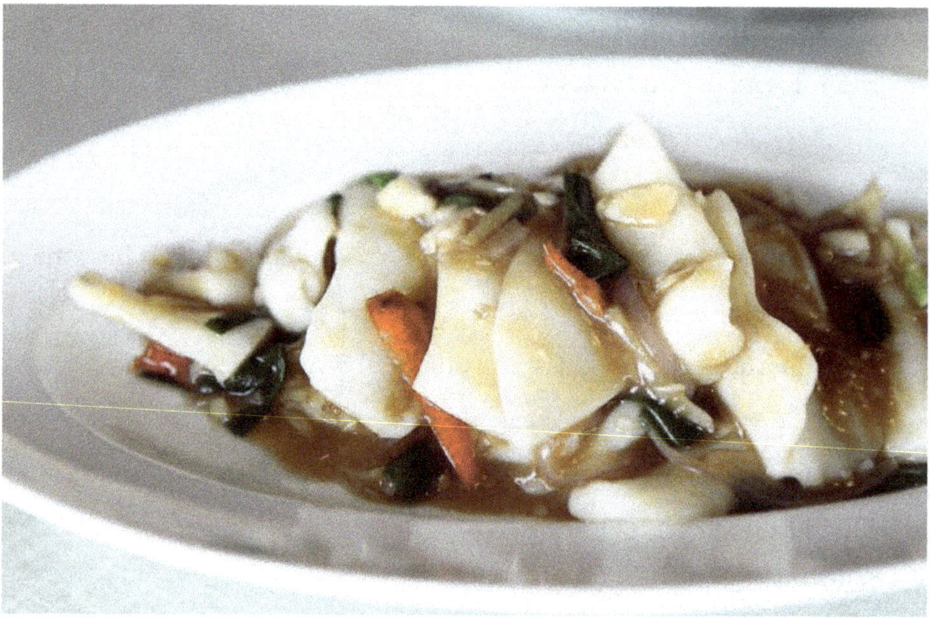

# Stuffed Squid

Preparation Time: 14 minutes | Cooking Time: 20 minutes | Servings:

**Ingredients:**

14-ounces dashi stock

4 squid, tentacles separated and chopped

1 cup cauliflower rice, cooked

2 tablespoons sake

1 tablespoon mirin

1 teaspoon Truvia

4 tablespoons soy sauce

**Directions:**

In a bowl, mix cauliflower rice, tentacles, stuff the squid with the mix.

Place the stuffed squid into your Pressure Pot, add the soy sauce, Truvia, mirin, sake, stir and cover.

Cook on high for 15-minutes.

Release pressure fast, divide squid between plates.

Serve warm!

**Nutrition:**

Calories 223, Fat 7g, Fiber 1g, Carbs 9g, Protein 29g.

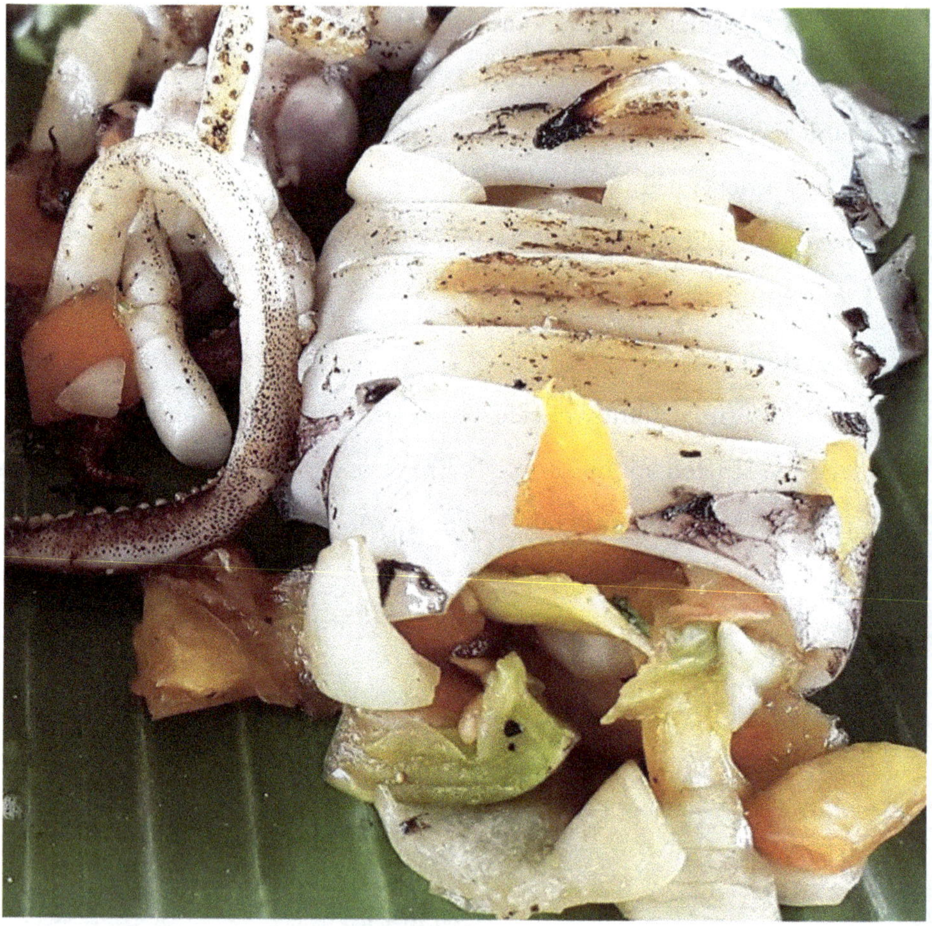

## Seafood Masala

Preparation Time: 14 minutes | Cooking Time: 15 minutes | Servings: 4

**Ingredients:**

1 ½ tablespoon red chili powder

17-ounces squid

¼ teaspoon mustard seeds

1 small ginger piece, grated

3 tablespoons olive oil

4 garlic cloves, minced

5 small coconut pieces, shredded

¼ teaspoon turmeric

2 cups of water

Salt and black pepper to taste

**Directions:**

In your Pressure Pot, mix the chili powder, squid, turmeric, water, salt, pepper, and cook on high for 15-minutes.

In your food processor, mix ginger with garlic, ginger, coconut, cumin, and pulse. Heat a pan with the oil over medium-high heat.

Add the mustard seeds, and toast them for 2-minutes and remove them from heat.

Release the pressure on the Pressure Pot naturally for 10-minutes. Transfer the squid and its liquid to the pan with mustard seeds.

Add the coconut paste as well.

Cook for a few minutes divides among serving plates.

Serve warm!

**Nutrition:**

Calories 216, Fat 6g, Fiber 1g, Carbs 15g, Protein 23g.

# Cream of Butternut Squash & Ginger Soup

Preparation Time: 5 Minutes | Cooking Time: 25 Minutes | Servings:4

**Ingredients:**

1 teaspoon extra-virgin olive oil

1 large Onion, roughly chopped

1 sprig of Sage

4-pound butternut squash, diced

½" piece of fresh ginger, minced

¼ teaspoon nutmeg

salt and pepper

4 cups vegetable stock

½ cup Toasted salty Pumpkin Seeds, to serve

**Directions:**

In your Pressure Pot, sauté onion with salt, pepper, and sage until softened.

Remove the onion mixture to a bowl and add squash cubes to the pot; sauté for 10 minutes and then add in the remaining ingredients including onion mixture.

Lock lid and cook on high pressure for 15 minutes; release pressure naturally and then discard sage.

Using an immersion blender, blend the mixture until smooth and serve garnished with toasted salt pumpkin seeds.

**Nutrition:**

Calories 323, Total Fats 9.6g, Carbs 59.7g, Protein 9.2g, Dietary Fiber 10.6g.

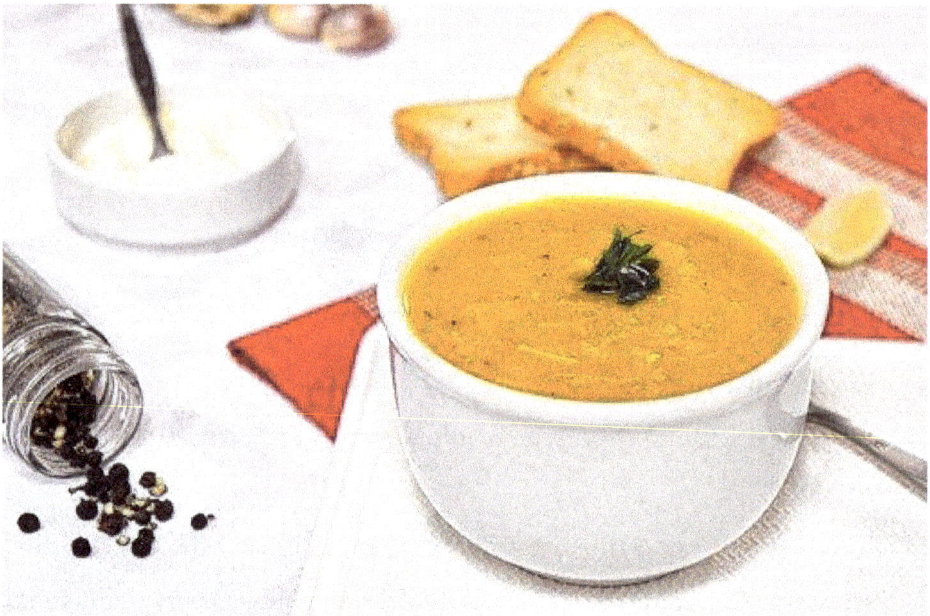

# Tasty Mushroom Coconut Milk Soup

Preparation Time: 10 Minutes | Cooking Time: 20 Minutes | Servings:4

**Ingredients:**

1 ½ pounds mushroom, trimmed

1 clove garlic, minced

2 red onions, chopped

4 cups vegetable stock

2 cups of coconut milk

1 tablespoon fresh thyme

1/8 teaspoon sea salt

Thyme sprigs

1/8 teaspoon pepper

**Directions:**

Grill the mushrooms, turning frequently, for about 5 minutes or until charred and tender; set aside.

In an Pressure Pot, sauté red onion in a splash of water. Stir in vegetable stock and cook for a few minutes.

Add the remaining ingredients and lock the lid; cook on high pressure for 3 minutes and then release the pressure naturally. Transfer the mixture to a blender and blend until very smooth.

Serve garnished with thyme sprigs.

**Nutrition:**

Calories 338, Total Fats 29.2g, Carbs 18.1g, Protein 8.8g, Dietary Fiber 5.8g.

# Tapioca Cold Fruit Soup

Preparation Time: 5 Minutes | Cooking Time: 20 minutes + chilling time | Servings: 4

**Ingredients:**

½ cup granulated sugar

4 tbsp tapioca

1 cup peach juice

2 apricots, cored and chopped

1 ½ cups raspberry juice

2 cups raspberries

1 cup strawberries, halved

1 cup blueberries

**Directions:**

In the inner pot, combine sugar, 1 cup water, tapioca, peach juice, and apricots. Seal the lid, select Manual/Pressure Cook on High, and set the time to 3 minutes. After cooking, perform a natural pressure release for 10 minutes. Unlock the lid.

Stir in raspberry juice, raspberries, strawberries, and blueberries. Spoon soup into serving bowls, allow cooling. Then chill in the refrigerator for 45 minutes to 1 hour.

Serve chilled.

**Nutrition:**

Calories 243, Carbs 61g, Fat 1g, Protein 2g.

# Cheesy Asparagus Soup

Preparation Time: 5 Minutes | Cooking Time: 30 minutes | Servings: 4

**Ingredients:**

1 onion, chopped

2 tbsp butter

1 carrot, sliced

4 cups chicken broth

1 cup milk

1 ½ pounds asparagus, chopped

1 cup half-and-half

2 cups shredded Cheddar cheese

Salt and black pepper to taste

**Directions:**

Set your Pressure Pot to Sauté mode and melt the butter. Cook the onion, asparagus, and carrot for 3 minutes, until tender. Pour in the chicken broth. Seal the lid, select Manual/Pressure Cook mode on High, and set the time to 8 minutes.

When done, perform a natural pressure release for 10 minutes, then a quick pressure release to let out the remaining steam. Stir in milk, half-and-half, and cheddar cheese until the cheese has melted.

Season with salt and pepper. Serve.

**Nutrition:**

Calories 202, Carbs 23g, Fat 10g, Protein 9g.

# Chili & Basil Tomato Soup

Preparation Time: 5 Minutes | Cooking Time: 20 minutes | Servings: 4

**Ingredients:**

3 lb tomatoes, peeled, chopped, with juice

1 onion, chopped

½ tsp chili flakes

1 cup chicken broth

Salt to taste

1 ½ cups milk

½ cup crème fraiche

2 tbsp basil, chopped

Salt and black pepper to taste

**Directions:**

In your Pressure Pot, add tomatoes, chicken broth, and salt. Seal the lid, select Manual/Pressure Cook on High, and set the cooking time to 5 minutes. When done, perform a quick pressure release.

Add in milk and crème and stir. Transfer to a food processor and puree the soup until smooth.

Return to the pot, press Sauté and stir until heated through about 5 minutes.

Sprinkle with chili flakes and basil to serve.

**Nutrition:**

Calories 287, Carbs 22g, Fat 14g, Protein 17g.

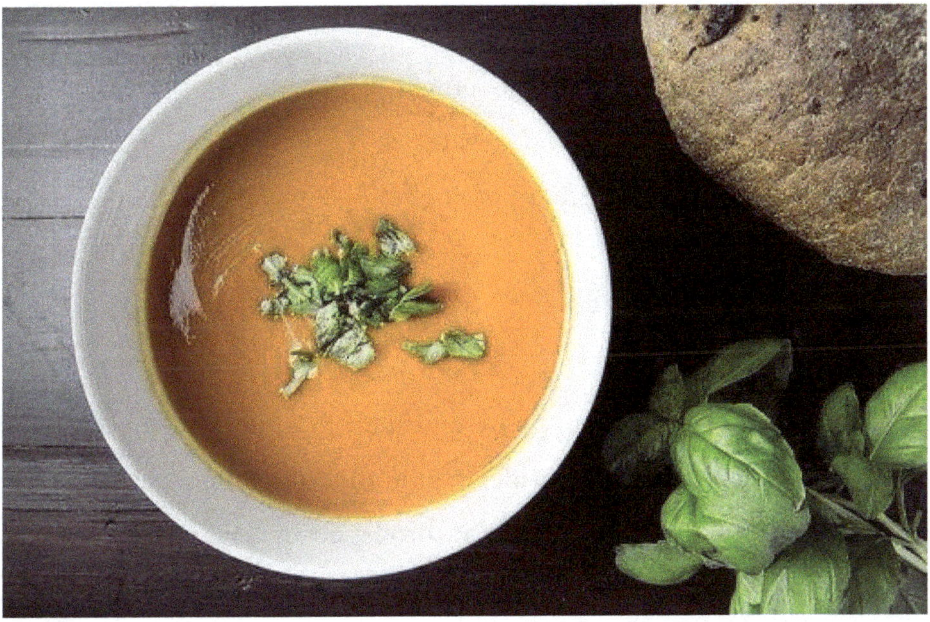

# Delicious Bacon & Bean Soup

Preparation Time: 5 Minutes | Cooking Time: 50 minutes | Servings: 4

**Ingredients:**

3 tbsp butter

1 onion, finely chopped

1 cup finely chopped fennel bulb

2 carrots, finely chopped

2 garlic cloves, minced

1-pound dried beans, soaked overnight

4 cups chicken broth

2 slices smoked bacon, chopped

2 tsp ground cumin

Salt and black pepper to taste

**Directions:**

Set your Pressure Pot to Sauté and melt the butter. Cook bacon for 5 minutes, until crispy. Set aside. Add in onion, fennel, carrots, and garlic, and sauté for 5 minutes. Pour in broth, beans, cumin, and salt. Stir to combine.

Seal the lid, select Manual/Pressure Cook on High, and set the time to 25 minutes. When done, perform a natural pressure release for 10 minutes. Unlock the lid and ladle soup in individual bowls. Top with reserved bacon to serve.

**Nutrition:**

Calories 229, Carbs 20g, Fat 15g, Protein 9g.

# Cream of Butter Squash

Preparation Time: 5 Minutes | Cooking Time: 25 minutes | Servings: 4

**Ingredients:**

2 pounds butter squash, peeled and cubed

2 sprigs parsley, chopped

1 onion, chopped

¼ tsp cumin

½-inch piece ginger, peeled and sliced

4 cups vegetable stock

½ cup sour cream

½ cup pumpkin seeds toasted, for garnish

Salt and black pepper to taste

2 tbsp olive oil + some for drizzling

**Directions:**

Set your Pressure Pot to Sauté and warm olive oil. Add onion, parsley, salt, and pepper, and sauté until the onion is soft. Place in butter squash and brown for 5 minutes, stirring often. Put in ginger, cumin, and vegetable stock, and stir.

Seal the lid, select Manual/Pressure Cook, cook for 10 minutes on High. When done, perform a quick pressure release. Pour mixture in a blender and puree until smooth. Stir in sour cream. Serve garnished with pumpkin seeds, and a drizzle of olive oil.

**Nutrition:**

Calories 276, Carbs 25g, Fat 18g, Protein 9g.

# Salmon and Black Olives Mix

Preparation time: 5 minutes | Cooking Time: 15 minutes | Servings: 4

**Ingredients:**

1 pound salmon fillets, boneless, skinless, and cubed

1 cup black olives, pitted and chopped

1 cup kalamata olives, pitted and chopped

2 garlic cloves, minced

1 tablespoon olive oil

A pinch of salt and black pepper

¼ cup chicken stock

1 tablespoon parsley, chopped

**Directions:**

Set the Pressure Pot on Sauté mode, add the oil, heat it, add the fish, and sear for 2 minutes on each side.

Add the rest of the ingredients, put the lid on, and cook on High for 10 minutes.

Release the pressure fast for 5 minutes, divide everything between plates and serve.

**Nutrition:**

Calories 261, fat 17.6g, fiber 2.2g, carbs 4.8g, protein 22.5g.

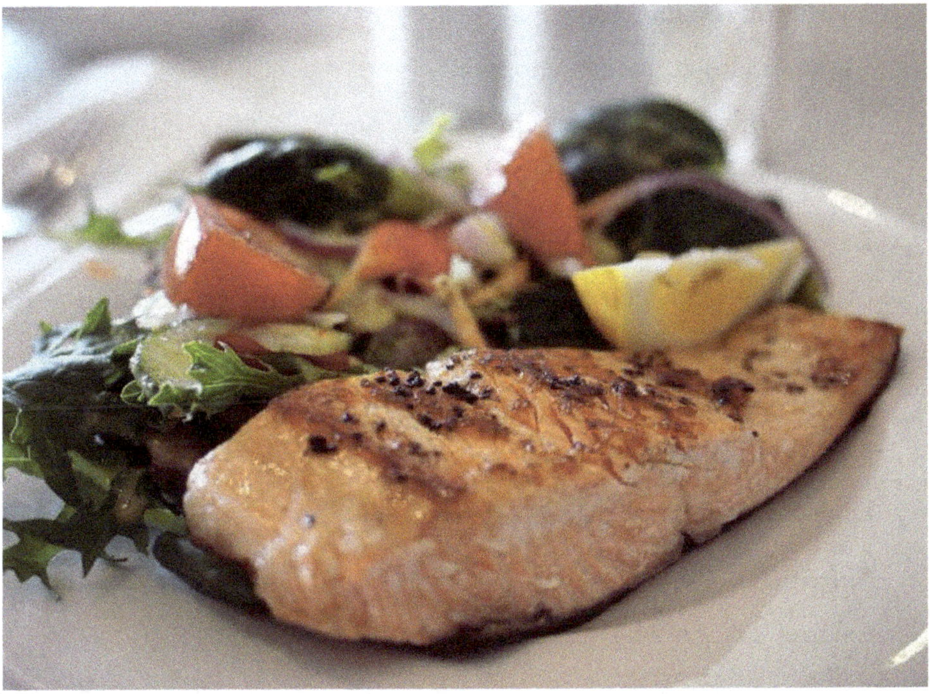

# Coriander Cod Mix

Preparation time: 5 minutes | Cooking Time: 15 minutes | Servings: 4

**Ingredients:**

4 cod fillets, boneless and skinless

1 cup coconut cream

2 spring onions, sliced

2 garlic cloves, minced

1 tablespoons coriander, chopped

A pinch of salt and black pepper

2 tablespoons lime juice

**Directions:**

In your Pressure Pot, combine the trout with the cream and the rest of the ingredients.

Put the lid on, and cook on High for 15 minutes.

Release the pressure fast for 5 minutes.

Divide everything between plates and serve.

**Nutrition:**

Calories 297, fat 24.3g, fiber 1.6g, carbs 5.4g, protein 17.6g.

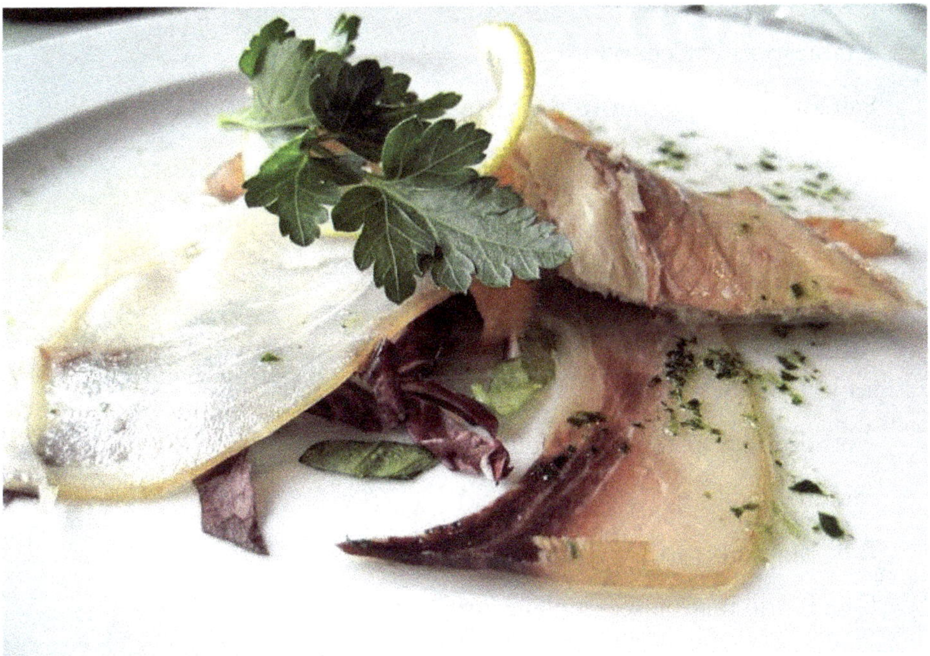

# Cod and Zucchinis

Preparation time: 5 minutes | Cooking Time: 15 minutes | Servings: 4

**Ingredients:**

4 cod fillets, boneless and skinless

2 zucchinis, sliced

1 tablespoon avocado oil

2 garlic cloves, minced

1 tablespoon sweet paprika

Salt and black pepper to the taste

1 tablespoon parsley, chopped

½ cup veggie stock

**Directions:**

Set the Pressure Pot on Sauté mode, add the oil, heat it, add the garlic and sauté for 2 minutes.

Add the rest of the ingredients , put the lid on, and cook on High for 12 minutes.

Release the pressure naturally for 5 minutes.

Divide the mix between plates and serve.

**Nutrition:**

Calories 182, fat 10.4g, fiber 1.9g, carbs 6.2g, protein 17.5g.

## Paprika Trout

Preparation time: 5 minutes | Cooking Time: 12 minutes | Servings: 4

### Ingredients:

4 trout fillets, boneless and skinless

½ cup chicken stock

A pinch of salt and black pepper

½ teaspoon oregano, dried

2 teaspoons sweet paprika

1 tablespoon chives, chopped

### Directions:

In your Pressure Pot, combine the trout with the rest of the ingredients, put the lid on, and cook on High for 12 minutes.

Release the pressure fast for 5 minutes.

Divide the mix between plates and serve.

### Nutrition:

Calories 132, fat 5.5g, fiber 0.5g, carbs 0.9g, protein 16.8g.

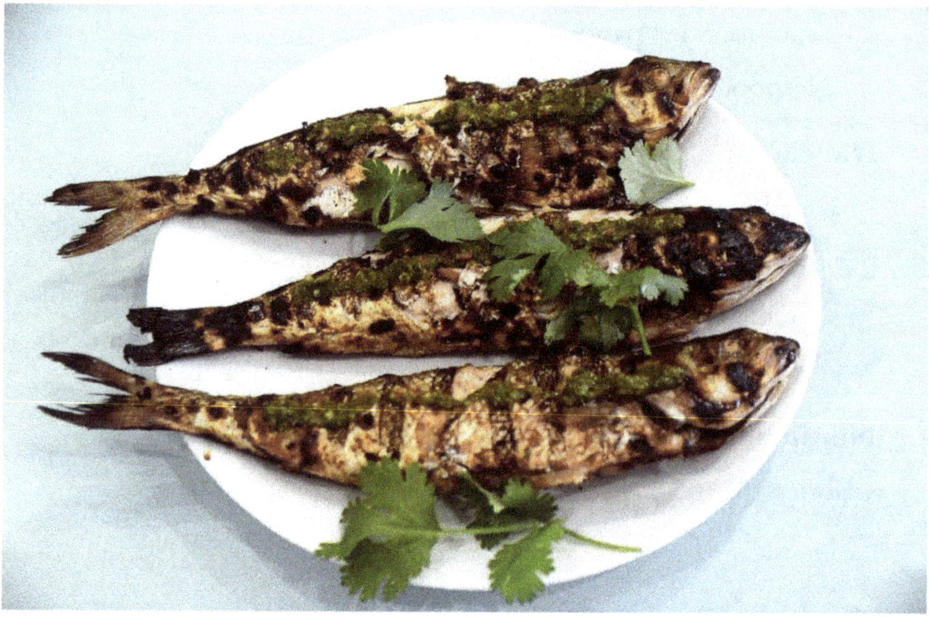

# Lime Shrimp

Preparation time: 5minutes | Cooking Time: 8 minutes | Servings: 4

**Ingredients:**

1-pound shrimp, peeled and deveined

Zest of 1 lime, grated

Juice of 1 lime

1 cup chicken stock

¼ cup cilantro, chopped

A pinch of salt and black pepper

**Directions:**

In your Pressure Pot, combine the shrimp with the rest of the ingredients, put the lid on, and cook on High for 8 minutes.

Release the pressure fast for 5 minutes.

Divide the shrimp between plates and serve with a side salad.

**Nutrition:**

Calories 138, fat 3.8g, fiber 0g, carbs 2g, protein 26g.

# Trout and Radishes

Preparation time: 5 minutes | Cooking Time: 12 minutes | Servings: 4

**Ingredients:**

4 trout fillets, boneless and skinless

A pinch of salt and black pepper

1 tablespoon parsley, chopped

2 tablespoons tomato passata

2 cups red radishes, sliced

**Directions:**

In your Pressure Pot, combine all the ingredients, put the lid on, and cook on High for 12 minutes.

Release the pressure fast for 5 minutes.

Divide everything between plates and serve.

**Nutrition:**

Calories 129, fat 5.3g, fiber 1.1g, carbs 2.5g, protein 17g.

# Cod and Broccoli

Preparation time: 5 minutes | Cooking Time: 15 minutes | Servings: 4

**Ingredients:**

4 cod fillets, boneless and skinless

A pinch of salt and black pepper

1-pound broccoli florets

2 tablespoon tomato passata

1 cup chicken stock

1 tablespoon cilantro, chopped

**Directions:**

In your Pressure Pot, combine all the ingredients, put the lid on, and cook on High for 15 minutes.

Release the pressure fast for 5 minutes.

Divide the mix between plates and serve.

**Nutrition:**

Calories 197, fat 10g, fiber 3.1g, carbs 4.3g, protein 19.4g.

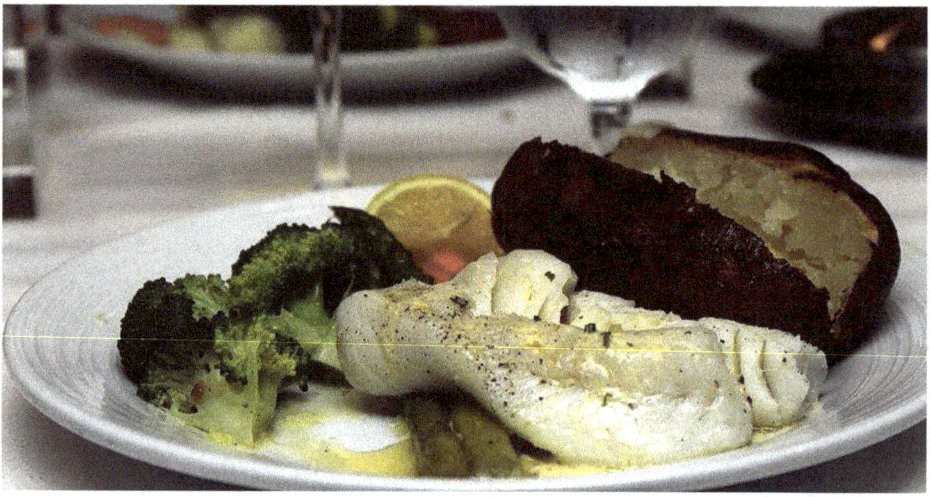

# Rosemary Trout and Cauliflower

Preparation time: 10 minutes | Cooking Time: 15 minutes | Servings: 4

**Ingredients:**

4 trout fillets, boneless and skinless

½ cup veggie stock

2 garlic cloves, minced

2 cups cauliflower florets

1 tablespoon avocado oil

A pinch of salt and black pepper

1 tablespoon rosemary, chopped

**Directions:**

Set the Pressure Pot on Sauté mode, add the oil, heat it, add the garlic and sauté for 2 minutes.

Add the rest of the ingredients, put the lid on, and cook on High for 13 minutes.

Release the pressure naturally for 10 minutes, divide the mix between plates and serve.

**Nutrition:**

Calories 140, fat 5.9g, fiber 1.8g, carbs 3.9g, protein 17.7g.

# Cinnamon Cod Mix

Preparation time: 5 minutes | Cooking Time: 12 minutes | Servings: 4

**Ingredients:**

4 cod fillets, boneless and skinless

1 tablespoon cinnamon powder

1 cup cherry tomatoes, cubed

Juice of ½ lemon

½ cup veggie stock

A pinch of salt and black pepper

1 tablespoon cilantro, chopped

**Directions:**

In your Pressure Pot, mix the fish with the rest of the ingredients, put the lid on, and cook on High for 12 minutes.

Release the pressure fast for 5 minutes, divide everything between plates and serve.

**Nutrition:**

Calories 162, fat 9.6g, fiber 0.3g, carbs 3g, protein 16.5g.

# Thai Pork Treat

Preparation Time: 5 minutes | Cooking Time: 35 minutes

Serving: 2

**Ingredients:**

1 tablespoon Thai curry paste

½ pound pork meat, boneless, sliced

½ cup of coconut milk

¼ cup of water

**Directions:**

Take your Pressure Pot and place it over a dry kitchen platform.

Open the lid and add the above-mentioned ingredients. Stir the ingredients gently to combine.

Lock the top lid and make sure that the valve is sealed properly.

Select "Manual" cooking function. Set the cooking time to 35 minutes.

Your Pressure Pot will start building the pressure and begin the cooking cycle after a sufficient level of pressure is reached.

After the cooking time is over, press the "Cancel" setting, and then press "NPR" for the natural release of the internal pressure. It takes around 10 minutes to release the pressure naturally.

Open the top lid and transfer the curry to your serving bowls.

Serve and enjoy the recipe.

**Nutrition:**

Calories 302, Total Carbohydrates 9g, Fiber 1g, Saturated Fat 12g, Trans Fat 0, Protein 25g, Sodium 412g.

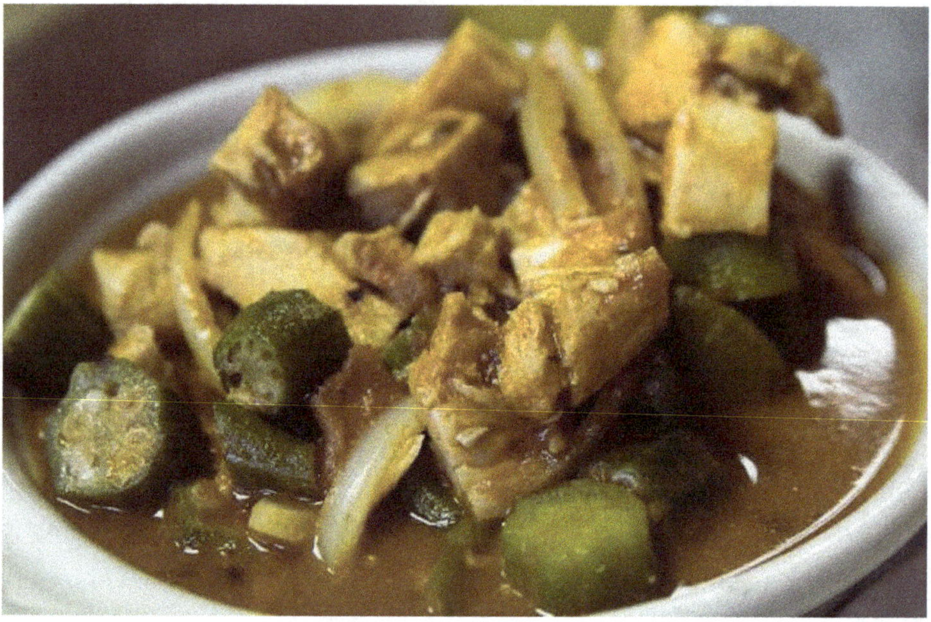

# Sausage-Stuffed Mushrooms

Preparation Time: 10 minutes | Cooking Time: 45 minutes

Serving: 2

**Ingredients:**

½ cup marinara sauce

½ cup ricotta cheese

2 large Portobello mushrooms

6 oz. pork sausage, minced

½ cup mozzarella cheese, shredded

¼ cup parsley (thoroughly chopped

**Directions:**

Stuff each mushroom cap with the pork sausage mince.

Add the ricotta cheese over the sausages and make a dent in the center.

Pour the marinara sauce into the dent.

Add the mozzarella cheese on top.

Take your Pressure Pot and place it over a dry kitchen platform.

Open the lid and pour some water into the pot.

Arrange a steaming basket inside.

Place the mushrooms into the basket

Lock the top lid and make sure that the valve is sealed properly.

Select "Manual" cooking function. Set the cooking time to 25 minutes.

Your Pressure Pot will start building the pressure and begin the cooking cycle after a sufficient level of pressure is reached.

After the cooking time is over, press the "Cancel" setting, and then press "NPR" for the natural release of the internal pressure. It takes around 10 minutes to release the pressure naturally.

Open the top lid and remove the stuffed mushrooms.

Serve and enjoy the recipe.

**Nutrition:**

Calories 567, Total Carbohydrates 26g, Fiber 7g, Saturated Fat 22g, Trans Fat 0g, Protein 35g, Sodium 1356g.

CPSIA information can be obtained
at www.ICGtesting.com
Printed in the USA
BVHW091127210621
610125BV00004B/912

9 781803 175256